NATURAL
REMEDIES FOR
ARTHRITIS

Herbal Remedies and Natural Medicine for All(NATURAL CURE AND REMEDIES FOR ARTHRITIS)

By

Dr. Mary D. Anna

DISCLAIMER

The information provided in this book, "Natural Remedies for Arthritis," is intended for general informational purposes only. It is not intended as a substitute for professional medical advice, diagnosis, or treatment. Always seek the advice of your physician or other qualified health provider with any questions you may have regarding a medical condition.

The author and publisher of this book have made every effort to ensure that the information provided is accurate and up-to-date at the time of publication. However, they make no representations or warranties of any kind, express or implied, about the completeness, accuracy, reliability, suitability, or availability of the information contained herein.

The remedies and techniques described in this book are based on the author's research and personal experience and may not be suitable for everyone. Individual results may vary, and the effectiveness of natural remedies for arthritis may depend on various factors, including but not limited to, the severity of the condition, individual health status, and adherence to the suggested guidelines.

While this book aims to provide valuable insights and information on natural remedies for arthritis, readers are encouraged to use their discretion and consult with a qualified healthcare professional before making any decisions regarding their health and well-being.

TABLE OF CONTENTS

INTRODUCTION

Arthritis, derived from the Greek words "arthron" meaning joint and "itis" meaning inflammation, is a condition characterized by inflammation and stiffness in the joints. It affects millions of people worldwide, making it one of the most prevalent chronic health conditions. There are several types of arthritis, each with its own unique characteristics and impact on the body. Among the most common types are osteoarthritis, rheumatoid arthritis, and gout. Understanding the different types of arthritis is essential for proper diagnosis and management.

Osteoarthritis, often referred to as "wear and tear" arthritis, is the most common form of arthritis, particularly among older adults. It occurs when the protective cartilage that cushions the ends of bones wears down over time, leading to pain, stiffness, and decreased mobility in the affected joints. Osteoarthritis commonly affects weight-bearing joints such as the knees, hips, and spine, but it can also occur in the hands and fingers.

Rheumatoid arthritis, on the other hand, is an autoimmune disease in which the body's immune system mistakenly attacks the synovium, the lining of the membranes that surround the joints. This results in inflammation, joint damage, and systemic symptoms such as fatigue and fever. Unlike osteoarthritis, rheumatoid arthritis can affect people of all ages and often leads to more severe joint deformities if left untreated.

Gout is another type of arthritis characterized by sudden and severe attacks of pain, redness, and swelling in the joints, particularly the big toe. It is caused by the accumulation of uric acid crystals in the joints, leading to inflammation and intense pain. Gout attacks can be triggered by certain foods, alcohol, obesity, and other factors, and they often occur intermittently over time.

The prevalence of arthritis is staggering, with millions of people worldwide living with this chronic condition. According to the World Health Organization (WHO), arthritis affects over 350 million people globally, making it a leading cause of disability and reduced quality of life. Its impact extends beyond physical discomfort, affecting mental health, social relationships, and overall well-being.

The symptoms of arthritis can vary depending on the type and severity of the condition, but common signs include joint pain, stiffness, swelling, and decreased range of motion. These symptoms can range from mild to debilitating, affecting everyday activities such as walking, climbing stairs, and even holding objects. In osteoarthritis, joint pain and stiffness are typically worse after periods of inactivity or overuse, whereas rheumatoid arthritis symptoms may be more persistent and accompanied by systemic manifestations like fatigue and morning stiffness.

Living with arthritis can be challenging, but early diagnosis and appropriate management strategies can help alleviate symptoms and improve quality of life. Treatment options may include medication, physical therapy, lifestyle modifications, and in some cases, surgery. It is essential for individuals with arthritis to work closely with healthcare professionals to develop a personalized treatment plan that addresses their unique needs and goals.

In conclusion, arthritis is a complex and prevalent condition that affects millions of people worldwide. By understanding the different types of arthritis, recognizing common symptoms, and seeking appropriate medical care, individuals can better manage their condition and lead fulfilling lives. Education, awareness, and support are key to empowering individuals living with arthritis to navigate the challenges they face and live well despite their diagnosis.

Understanding Arthritis: Exploring Causes, Diagnosis, and Complications

Arthritis is a complex and multifaceted condition that can significantly impact an individual's quality of life. To effectively manage and treat arthritis, it's crucial to understand its underlying causes, methods of diagnosis, and potential complications. In this comprehensive discussion, we'll explore these aspects of arthritis in a human tone, providing valuable insights for individuals affected by this condition.

Causes of Arthritis:
Arthritis can arise from a combination of genetic, age-related, lifestyle, and environmental factors. While the exact cause of many types of arthritis remains unknown, researchers have identified several contributing factors:

Genetics: Family history plays a significant role in the development of certain types of arthritis, such as rheumatoid arthritis and ankylosing spondylitis. Individuals with a family history of arthritis may have a higher risk of developing the condition themselves due to inherited genetic predispositions.

Age: The risk of developing arthritis increases with age, particularly osteoarthritis. As the body's joints undergo wear and tear over time, the protective cartilage that cushions the bones may gradually deteriorate, leading to joint pain and stiffness.

Lifestyle Factors: Certain lifestyle choices, such as obesity, sedentary behavior, and repetitive joint stress, can contribute to the development and progression of arthritis. Excess weight puts added strain on the joints, particularly the knees, hips, and spine, increasing the risk of osteoarthritis. Additionally, occupations or activities that involve repetitive movements or joint overuse may accelerate joint damage and inflammation.

Environmental Factors: Environmental factors, including exposure to toxins, infectious agents, and pollutants, may also play a role in triggering arthritis, particularly autoimmune forms such as rheumatoid arthritis. While the specific environmental triggers for arthritis remain unclear, ongoing research aims to uncover potential links between environmental factors and the development of the condition.

Diagnosis of Arthritis:

Diagnosing arthritis typically involves a combination of medical history, physical examinations, imaging tests, and laboratory tests. Healthcare professionals use these diagnostic tools to evaluate symptoms, assess joint function, and confirm the presence of arthritis. Here's an overview of the diagnostic process:

Medical History: Healthcare providers will begin by conducting a thorough medical history, discussing symptoms, family history of arthritis, and any underlying health conditions or previous injuries that may contribute to joint pain and inflammation.

Physical Examination: A physical examination allows healthcare providers to assess joint function, range of motion, swelling, and tenderness. They may also perform specific maneuvers to elicit pain or instability in the affected joints.

Imaging Tests: Imaging tests, such as X-rays, magnetic resonance imaging (MRI), and computed tomography (CT) scans, can provide detailed images of the joints, allowing healthcare providers to visualize structural abnormalities, joint damage, and signs of arthritis.

Laboratory Tests: Blood tests, including tests for inflammatory markers such as C-reactive protein (CRP) and erythrocyte sedimentation rate (ESR), may be ordered to assess inflammation levels in the body. Additionally, antibody tests, such as rheumatoid factor and anti-cyclic citrullinated peptide (anti-CCP) antibodies, may help diagnose autoimmune forms of arthritis like rheumatoid arthritis.

Complications of Arthritis:
Arthritis can lead to various complications that affect joint function, mobility, and overall quality of life. Some common complications associated with arthritis include:

Joint Damage: Persistent inflammation and joint erosion can lead to irreversible damage to the cartilage, bones, and surrounding tissues, resulting in joint deformities, instability, and limited mobility. Severe joint damage may require surgical intervention, such as joint replacement surgery, to restore function and alleviate pain.

Disability: As arthritis progresses, individuals may experience increasing pain, stiffness, and difficulty performing daily activities, ultimately leading to disability. Joint deformities, muscle weakness, and joint instability can significantly impair mobility and independence, impacting one's ability to work, engage in social activities, and maintain a fulfilling lifestyle.

Reduced Quality of Life: Arthritis can have a profound impact on overall quality of life, affecting physical, emotional, and social well-being. Chronic pain, fatigue, and functional limitations can lead to feelings of frustration, depression, and isolation. Additionally, managing arthritis may require ongoing medical treatment, lifestyle modifications, and adaptations to daily routines, which can add to the burden of the condition.

Understanding the causes, diagnosis, and potential complications of arthritis is essential for effectively managing and treating this chronic condition. By addressing contributing factors, diagnosing arthritis accurately, and addressing complications early, individuals can take proactive steps to minimize the impact of arthritis on their lives and improve overall well-being. Empowered with knowledge and support from healthcare professionals, individuals affected by arthritis can navigate their journey with confidence and resilience, finding ways to thrive despite the challenges they may face.

When it comes to managing arthritis, a variety of conventional treatment options are available to help individuals alleviate pain, reduce inflammation, and improve joint function. These treatments encompass medications, physical therapy, and surgical interventions, each playing a crucial role in enhancing the quality of life for those affected by arthritis.

Medications:
Medications are often the first line of defense in arthritis management, aiming to relieve pain and inflammation while slowing down the progression of the disease. Some commonly prescribed medications for arthritis include:

1. Analgesics: Pain relievers, such as acetaminophen, help alleviate mild to moderate joint pain without reducing inflammation. They are often recommended for individuals with osteoarthritis who experience primarily pain-related symptoms.

2. Nonsteroidal Anti-inflammatory Drugs (NSAIDs): NSAIDs, including ibuprofen,

naproxen, and aspirin, are commonly used to reduce pain and inflammation associated with arthritis. They work by blocking the production of prostaglandins, chemicals that contribute to inflammation and pain in the joints. NSAIDs are particularly beneficial for individuals with inflammatory forms of arthritis, such as rheumatoid arthritis.

3. Disease-Modifying Antirheumatic Drugs (DMARDs): DMARDs, such as methotrexate, hydroxychloroquine, and sulfasalazine, are used to slow down the progression of autoimmune forms of arthritis, such as rheumatoid arthritis. They work by suppressing the overactive immune response that attacks the joints and causes inflammation and joint damage.

It's essential for individuals to work closely with their healthcare providers to determine the most appropriate medication regimen based on their specific type of arthritis, symptoms, and overall health status. Regular monitoring and adjustments to medication dosages may be necessary to achieve optimal pain relief and disease management.

Physical Therapy:
Physical therapy plays a crucial role in arthritis management by improving joint function, reducing pain, and enhancing mobility through targeted exercises and interventions. A physical therapist can design a customized treatment plan tailored to the individual's unique needs and goals, focusing on:

1. Joint Mobility and Flexibility: Range-of-motion exercises help improve joint flexibility and reduce stiffness, making it easier to perform daily activities with less pain and discomfort.

2. Muscle Strengthening: Strengthening exercises target the muscles surrounding the affected joints, providing stability and support to reduce joint strain and improve overall function.

3. Pain Management Techniques: Physical therapists may incorporate modalities such as heat therapy, cold therapy, ultrasound, and transcutaneous electrical nerve stimulation (TENS) to alleviate pain and inflammation in the joints.

4. Assistive Devices and Techniques: Physical therapists can recommend assistive devices, such as braces, splints, or orthotics, to support and protect the joints during daily activities. They may also teach individuals proper body mechanics and ergonomic techniques to minimize joint stress and prevent injury.

By participating in regular physical therapy sessions and adhering to prescribed exercise programs, individuals with arthritis can experience significant improvements in joint mobility, strength, and overall function, allowing them to maintain independence and enjoy a better quality of life.

Surgery:
In severe cases of arthritis where conservative treatments fail to provide adequate relief, surgical intervention may be necessary to repair damaged joints and alleviate pain. Some common surgical options for arthritis include:

1. Joint Replacement Surgery: Joint replacement surgery, such as total knee replacement, total hip replacement, or total

shoulder replacement, involves removing damaged joint surfaces and replacing them with artificial implants made of metal, plastic, or ceramic. This procedure can effectively relieve pain, improve joint function, and restore mobility for individuals with advanced arthritis.

2. Arthroscopic Surgery: Arthroscopic surgery is a minimally invasive procedure performed to diagnose and treat certain types of arthritis, such as osteoarthritis or rheumatoid arthritis, by removing damaged tissue, repairing cartilage defects, or smoothing rough joint surfaces. It may be recommended to relieve symptoms and delay the need for more extensive surgical interventions.

While surgery can offer significant benefits for individuals with severe arthritis, it's important to carefully weigh the risks and benefits with a healthcare provider and explore alternative treatment options before proceeding with surgery. Postoperative rehabilitation and ongoing monitoring are essential for optimizing surgical outcomes and ensuring long-term joint function and mobility.

Conventional treatments for arthritis encompass a range of modalities aimed at managing pain, reducing inflammation, and improving joint function. By combining medications, physical therapy, and surgical interventions as needed, individuals with arthritis can effectively manage their symptoms, slow down disease progression, and maintain an active and fulfilling lifestyle. It's essential for individuals to work closely with their healthcare providers to develop personalized treatment plans that address their unique needs and goals, empowering them to live well despite the challenges posed by arthritis.

Living with arthritis presents unique challenges, but making lifestyle modifications can significantly improve quality of life and help manage symptoms. By incorporating regular exercise, adopting a healthy diet, and implementing stress management techniques, individuals with arthritis can promote joint health, reduce inflammation, and enhance overall well-being.

Exercise: Regular exercise is essential for maintaining joint flexibility, muscle strength, and overall physical health for individuals with arthritis. While it may seem counterintuitive to move when joints are stiff and painful, engaging in appropriate exercises can actually help alleviate symptoms and improve joint function. Some beneficial exercises for arthritis include:

1. Low-Impact Activities: Activities such as walking, swimming, cycling, and water aerobics are gentle on the joints while providing cardiovascular benefits and promoting overall fitness. These low-impact exercises help

improve joint flexibility and range of motion without causing undue stress or strain.

2. Strength Training: Strength training exercises, using light weights or resistance bands, help strengthen the muscles surrounding the joints, providing stability and support. Strong muscles can help reduce joint pain and improve joint function, making daily activities easier to perform.

3. Flexibility and Range-of-Motion Exercises: Stretching and range-of-motion exercises help maintain or improve joint flexibility, reducing stiffness and preventing further joint deterioration. Incorporating gentle stretching routines into daily activities can help alleviate joint pain and improve mobility.

It's important for individuals with arthritis to start slowly and gradually increase the intensity and duration of their exercise routines under the guidance of a healthcare provider or physical therapist. Listening to the body and avoiding activities that exacerbate pain or discomfort is key to preventing injury and promoting long-term joint health.

Diet: The impact of diet on arthritis symptoms cannot be overstated, as certain foods can either contribute to inflammation or help alleviate it. Adopting a balanced diet rich in anti-inflammatory foods can help reduce joint pain and inflammation while promoting overall health. Some recommended dietary strategies for arthritis management include:

1. Incorporating Fruits and Vegetables: Fruits and vegetables are rich in vitamins, minerals, and antioxidants that help reduce inflammation and support joint health. Aim to include a variety of colorful fruits and vegetables in your diet, such as berries, leafy greens, citrus fruits, and cruciferous vegetables.

2. Choosing Whole Grains: Whole grains, such as brown rice, quinoa, oats, and barley, provide fiber and nutrients that help regulate inflammation and promote digestive health. Opt for whole grain options over refined grains to maximize their anti-inflammatory benefits.

3. Including Omega-3 Fatty Acids: Omega-3 fatty acids, found in fatty fish like salmon,

mackerel, and sardines, as well as in flaxseeds, chia seeds, and walnuts, have anti-inflammatory properties that can help reduce joint pain and stiffness. Incorporating omega-3-rich foods into your diet regularly can help support joint health and overall well-being.

4. Limiting Processed Foods and Added Sugars: Processed foods, sugary snacks, and beverages high in refined sugars can contribute to inflammation and exacerbate arthritis symptoms. Limiting intake of these foods and focusing on whole, nutrient-dense options can help manage inflammation and support overall health.

By making informed dietary choices and focusing on nutrient-rich, anti-inflammatory foods, individuals with arthritis can help alleviate symptoms and improve their overall well-being.

Stress Management:

Stress can exacerbate arthritis symptoms and contribute to increased pain and inflammation. Implementing stress management techniques can help individuals with arthritis better cope with their condition and improve their overall quality of life. Some effective stress-reduction techniques include:

1.   Meditation: Practicing   mindfulness meditation techniques, such as deep breathing exercises, guided imagery, or body scan meditation, can help calm the mind, reduce stress, and promote relaxation. Even just a few minutes of meditation each day can have a profound impact on stress levels and well-being.

2. Yoga: Yoga combines gentle stretching, breathing exercises, and mindfulness techniques to promote physical and mental relaxation. Regular practice of yoga can help improve flexibility, reduce muscle tension, and alleviate stress and anxiety associated with arthritis.

3. Deep Breathing Exercises: Deep breathing exercises, such as diaphragmatic breathing or progressive muscle relaxation, help activate the body's relaxation response, reducing stress levels and promoting a sense of calm and well-being. Taking a few moments each day to practice deep breathing can help manage arthritis-related stress and improve overall mental health.

4. Engaging in Hobbies and Activities: Engaging in enjoyable hobbies and activities, such as gardening, painting, or listening to music, can provide a welcome distraction from arthritis-related pain and stress. Finding activities that bring joy and fulfillment can help individuals with arthritis maintain a positive outlook and improve their overall quality of life.

In conclusion, making lifestyle modifications that prioritize regular exercise, a healthy diet, and stress management can play a significant role in managing arthritis symptoms and improving overall well-being. By incorporating these strategies into daily life, individuals with arthritis can take proactive steps to promote joint health, reduce inflammation, and enhance their quality of life. It's important to work closely with healthcare providers to develop personalized lifestyle plans that address individual needs and preferences, empowering individuals to live well despite the challenges of arthritis.

Natural Remedies for Arthritis: Exploring Herbal Remedies, Topical Treatments, and Alternative Therapies

In addition to conventional treatments, many individuals with arthritis seek relief through natural remedies and alternative therapies. While scientific evidence may vary for their effectiveness, some herbal remedies, topical treatments, and alternative therapies have shown promise in reducing inflammation and alleviating arthritis symptoms. Let's explore these natural approaches in more detail.

Herbal Remedies:

Herbs and supplements have been used for centuries in traditional medicine systems to alleviate pain and inflammation associated with arthritis. While research on their effectiveness is ongoing, several herbs and supplements have garnered attention for their potential benefits:

1. Turmeric: Turmeric, a spice derived from the Curcuma longa plant, contains a compound called curcumin, which exhibits anti-inflammatory and antioxidant properties. Studies suggest that turmeric may help reduce

inflammation and relieve joint pain in individuals with arthritis.

2. Ginger: Ginger is another herb with anti-inflammatory properties that may help alleviate arthritis symptoms. It contains compounds called gingerols and shogaols, which have been shown to reduce inflammation and inhibit the production of inflammatory chemicals in the body.

3. Fish Oil: Fish oil supplements, rich in omega-3 fatty acids, have been studied for their potential benefits in reducing inflammation and improving joint health in individuals with arthritis. Omega-3 fatty acids, particularly EPA and DHA, may help decrease joint stiffness and pain by reducing inflammation in the body.

While herbal remedies like turmeric, ginger, and fish oil show promise in managing arthritis symptoms, it's essential to consult with a healthcare provider before incorporating them into your treatment regimen, especially if you're taking medications or have underlying health conditions.

Topical Treatments:

Topical treatments, such as creams, gels, and patches, can provide localized pain relief for arthritis symptoms. These products typically contain active ingredients that help alleviate pain and inflammation when applied directly to the affected joints. Some commonly used topical treatments for arthritis include:

1. Capsaicin Cream: Capsaicin, derived from chili peppers, is a natural pain reliever that works by desensitizing nerve receptors and reducing pain signals to the brain. Capsaicin cream is often applied topically to the skin to relieve joint pain and stiffness associated with arthritis.

2. Menthol-Based Products: Menthol, a natural compound derived from mint plants, produces a cooling sensation when applied to the skin, which can help alleviate arthritis-related pain and discomfort. Menthol-based creams, gels, and patches are commonly used to provide temporary relief from joint pain and inflammation.

3. Arnica: Arnica, a herbaceous plant native to Europe and North America, has been used traditionally to treat bruises, sprains, and muscle soreness. Arnica-based creams and ointments may help reduce pain, swelling, and stiffness in individuals with arthritis when applied topically to affected joints.

While topical treatments can provide symptomatic relief for arthritis, it's important to follow the manufacturer's instructions and avoid applying them to broken or irritated skin. Additionally, topical treatments are generally considered safe when used as directed, but some individuals may experience skin irritation or allergic reactions, so it's essential to perform a patch test before widespread use.

Alternative Therapies:
In addition to herbal remedies and topical treatments, alternative therapies offer complementary approaches to managing arthritis symptoms and promoting overall well-being. These therapies focus on holistic healing and may help reduce pain, improve joint function, and enhance quality of life for

individuals with arthritis. Some popular alternative therapies for arthritis include:

1. Acupuncture: Acupuncture is a traditional Chinese medicine practice that involves inserting thin needles into specific points on the body to stimulate energy flow and promote healing. Studies suggest that acupuncture may help reduce arthritis-related pain and improve joint function by triggering the release of endorphins, the body's natural pain-relieving chemicals.

2. Massage Therapy: Massage therapy involves manipulating soft tissues and muscles to reduce tension, improve circulation, and alleviate pain. Therapeutic massage techniques, such as Swedish massage, deep tissue massage, and myofascial release, may help relax stiff muscles, reduce inflammation, and improve range of motion in individuals with arthritis.

3. Chiropractic Care: Chiropractic care focuses on spinal alignment and joint manipulation to restore proper joint function and alleviate pain. Chiropractors use hands-on techniques, such as spinal adjustments and mobilizations, to address

misalignments and improve nerve function, which may help reduce arthritis-related pain and stiffness.

While alternative therapies like acupuncture, massage therapy, and chiropractic care may offer symptomatic relief for arthritis, it's essential to consult with qualified practitioners and discuss treatment options with a healthcare provider to ensure safe and effective care. Integrating these therapies into a comprehensive treatment plan that includes conventional treatments and lifestyle modifications can help individuals with arthritis achieve optimal outcomes and improve their overall quality of life.

In conclusion, natural remedies and alternative therapies offer additional options for managing arthritis symptoms and promoting joint health. While scientific evidence may vary for their effectiveness, herbs, topical treatments, and alternative therapies have shown promise in reducing inflammation, alleviating pain, and improving overall well-being for individuals with arthritis. It's important to approach these treatments with caution, consult with healthcare providers, and integrate them into a comprehensive treatment plan tailored to individual needs and preferences. By exploring natural remedies and alternative therapies in conjunction with conventional treatments and lifestyle modifications, individuals with arthritis can take proactive steps toward managing their condition and enhancing their quality of life.

REMEDY ONE

Harnessing the Power of Turmeric: Nature's Anti-Inflammatory Hero for Arthritis Relief

In the realm of natural remedies for arthritis, few substances shine as brightly as turmeric. Renowned for its vibrant hue and rich flavor, this ancient spice boasts a potent compound called curcumin. Beyond its culinary allure, curcumin stands out for its remarkable anti-inflammatory properties, making turmeric a valuable ally in the fight against arthritis pain and inflammation.

Understanding Turmeric and Curcumin:
At the heart of turmeric's therapeutic prowess lies curcumin, a bioactive compound with a myriad of health benefits. Research suggests that curcumin exerts its anti-inflammatory effects by inhibiting various molecular pathways involved in inflammation. By modulating these pathways, curcumin helps to alleviate pain and stiffness associated with arthritis, offering a natural alternative to traditional pharmaceuticals.

The Science Behind Turmeric's Efficacy:
Numerous studies have delved into the mechanisms through which turmeric and curcumin exert their anti-inflammatory effects. One key pathway involves the inhibition of inflammatory enzymes, such as cyclooxygenase-2 (COX-2), which play a central role in the production of pro-inflammatory molecules. By blocking these enzymes, curcumin helps to dampen the inflammatory response, providing relief from arthritis symptoms.

Furthermore, curcumin has been shown to suppress the activity of nuclear factor-kappa B (NF-kB), a master regulator of inflammation. By inhibiting NF-kB, curcumin helps to downregulate the expression of genes involved in inflammation, thereby attenuating the inflammatory cascade.

Additionally, curcumin exhibits antioxidant properties, scavenging free radicals and reducing oxidative stress within the joints. This antioxidative action not only protects against cartilage degradation but also contributes to overall joint health and function.

Incorporating Turmeric into Your Routine:
Harnessing the benefits of turmeric for arthritis relief can be easily achieved through dietary supplementation or culinary exploration. Adding turmeric to your daily meals not only enhances flavor but also delivers a therapeutic dose of curcumin. Whether sprinkled onto roasted vegetables, stirred into curries, or brewed into a soothing tea, turmeric offers a versatile and delicious way to support joint health.

For those seeking a more concentrated dose of curcumin, supplements are readily available in various forms, including capsules, powders, and extracts. When choosing a supplement, opt for products standardized to contain high levels of curcuminoids, the active compounds in turmeric. Additionally, pairing turmeric with black pepper or piperine can enhance curcumin absorption, maximizing its therapeutic potential.

The Holistic Approach to Arthritis Management:
While turmeric holds promise as a natural remedy for arthritis, it is essential to adopt a

holistic approach to management. Incorporating other lifestyle modifications, such as regular exercise, stress management, and a balanced diet, can synergistically enhance the efficacy of turmeric in relieving arthritis symptoms.

Moreover, consulting with a healthcare professional is advisable before initiating any new treatment regimen, especially for individuals with pre-existing medical conditions or those taking medications that may interact with turmeric supplements.

In conclusion, turmeric stands as a beacon of hope for individuals grappling with the debilitating effects of arthritis. Through its potent anti-inflammatory and antioxidative properties, turmeric offers a natural and effective means of alleviating pain and improving joint function. By incorporating turmeric into your daily routine, whether through culinary exploration or dietary supplementation, you can harness the healing power of this golden spice and embark on a journey towards enhanced joint health and overall well-being.

REMEDY TWO

Exploring the Benefits of Omega-3 Fatty Acids for Arthritis Relief

When it comes to managing arthritis symptoms, exploring natural remedies can offer significant relief and support. One such remedy that has garnered attention for its potential benefits is omega-3 fatty acids. These essential fatty acids, commonly found in fatty fish like salmon, mackerel, and sardines, have been increasingly recognized for their ability to alleviate joint pain and stiffness, making them a valuable addition to any arthritis management plan.

Understanding Omega-3 Fatty Acids:
Omega-3 fatty acids are a type of polyunsaturated fat that play crucial roles in various bodily functions, including reducing inflammation. There are three primary forms of omega-3 fatty acids: alpha-linolenic acid (ALA), eicosapentaenoic acid (EPA), and docosahexaenoic acid (DHA). While ALA is primarily found in plant sources like flaxseeds, chia seeds, and walnuts, EPA and DHA are predominantly found in fatty fish.

The Anti-inflammatory Properties of Omega-3s: Inflammation is a key driver of arthritis symptoms, contributing to pain, swelling, and reduced mobility in affected joints. Omega-3 fatty acids have been shown to exert powerful anti-inflammatory effects in the body, helping to counteract the inflammatory processes that occur in arthritis.

Research Supporting Omega-3s for Arthritis Relief:
Numerous studies have investigated the potential benefits of omega-3 fatty acids for arthritis sufferers, with promising results. A systematic review published in the "Journal of Nutrition in Gerontology and Geriatrics" examined the effects of omega-3 supplementation on rheumatoid arthritis and found that it significantly reduced disease activity and joint tenderness.

Another study published in the Annals of the Rheumatic Diseases evaluated the impact of omega-3 fatty acids on patients with osteoarthritis and found that supplementation led to improvements in joint pain and function, particularly in individuals with moderate to severe symptoms.

Incorporating Omega-3s into Your Diet:
One of the most accessible ways to increase your intake of omega-3 fatty acids is by including fatty fish in your regular diet. Salmon, mackerel, sardines, and trout are all excellent sources of EPA and DHA. Aim to consume at least two servings of fatty fish per week to reap the benefits of omega-3s for arthritis relief.

If you're not a fan of fish or have dietary restrictions that prevent you from consuming seafood, you can still benefit from omega-3 supplementation. Fish oil capsules are widely available and provide a convenient way to ensure you're getting an adequate amount of these essential fatty acids in your diet. When choosing a fish oil supplement, opt for a high-quality product that has been tested for purity and potency.

Tips for Maximizing the Benefits of Omega-3s:
While incorporating omega-3 fatty acids into your diet can be beneficial for arthritis relief,

there are some tips to keep in mind to maximize their effectiveness:

1. Consistency is Key: To experience the full benefits of omega-3s, it's important to consume them regularly as part of a balanced diet. Aim for consistency in your intake of fatty fish or fish oil supplements to maintain steady levels of these essential fatty acids in your body.

2. Pair Omega-3s with Antioxidants: Combining omega-3 fatty acids with antioxidant-rich foods can enhance their anti-inflammatory effects. Consider incorporating fruits, vegetables, and spices like turmeric and ginger into your meals to complement the benefits of omega-3s for arthritis relief.

3. Monitor Your Symptoms: Keep track of your arthritis symptoms before and after incorporating omega-3s into your diet to gauge their effectiveness. Pay attention to changes in pain levels, joint stiffness, and overall mobility to determine whether omega-3s are contributing to symptom improvement.

4. Consult with Your Healthcare Provider: If you're considering adding omega-3 supplements to your arthritis management plan, it's a good idea to consult with your healthcare provider first. They can offer personalized recommendations based on your individual health status and any medications you may be taking.

Omega-3 fatty acids hold promise as a natural remedy for arthritis relief, thanks to their potent anti-inflammatory properties. Whether consumed through fatty fish or supplements, omega-3s can play a valuable role in managing joint pain and stiffness associated with arthritis. By incorporating these essential fatty acids into your diet and lifestyle, you can take proactive steps towards improving your overall joint health and quality of life.

REMEDY THREE

Ginger, frequently lauded for its culinary attraction, extends beyond conventional flavor improvement. Its unique repertory includes significant anti-inflammatory qualities, making it a formidable ally in the struggle against arthritic discomfort. Renowned for millennia in traditional medicine, ginger offers a comprehensive approach to reducing symptoms, acting as a beacon of solace amidst the struggles of controlling arthritis.

At the heart of ginger's medicinal effectiveness lies its diverse makeup of bioactive chemicals. Chief among these is gingerol, a phenolic substance endowed with potent anti-inflammatory and antioxidant capabilities. Through regulation of several inflammatory pathways in the body, gingerol provides a calming action on joints afflicted by arthritis. This multimodal approach not only curtails inflammation but also helps attenuate oxidative stress, therefore reinforcing the body's resilience against the degenerative consequences of arthritis.

Harnessing the advantages of ginger for arthritis treatment can take numerous forms, each filled with its distinct charm and efficiency. One such outlet is ginger tea, a time-honored treatment appreciated for its simplicity and efficiency. By steeping freshly grated ginger in hot water, one may unleash its medicinal essence, giving a fragrant infusion loaded with anti-inflammatory virtues. Consumed frequently, ginger tea is a comfortable ritual that relaxes both body and spirit, bringing reprieve from the unrelenting throes of arthritic agony.

Beyond the world of drinks, ginger readily integrates into culinary undertakings, complementing meals with its characteristic taste profile while simultaneously giving its healing touch. From stir-fries to soups, the use of fresh ginger not only tantalizes the taste senses but also gives a therapeutic component to meals. Its diverse nature allows for creative exploration, encouraging folks to explore the broad culinary terrain while reaping the advantages of ginger's anti-inflammatory richness.

Moreover, ginger's effect goes beyond its direct ingestion, penetrating the domain of holistic remedies and alternative medicine. In the field of aromatherapy, ginger essential oil appears as a formidable cure, capable of offering focused comfort to achy joints and fatigued muscles. Diluted with a carrier oil and gently rubbed into problematic regions, ginger essential oil penetrates deep into tissues, unwinding tension and instilling a sense of vibrancy. This comprehensive approach to arthritis care transcends the physical domain, establishing a harmonic harmony between mind, body, and spirit.

In essence, ginger appears as a beacon of light within the maze of arthritis therapy, giving a natural and comprehensive approach to reducing symptoms. Its varied advantages, spanning from anti-inflammatory power to culinary variety, emphasize its relevance as a strong partner in the quest for relief. By adding ginger into daily rituals and culinary exploits, individuals may start on a path of empowerment, reclaiming control over their well-being and enjoying a life enhanced by the healing touch of nature's richness.

REMEDY FOUR

The Healing Touch: Exploring the Benefits of Massage Therapy for Arthritis Management

Arthritis, a medical condition defined by inflammation and stiffness in the joints, can drastically influence one's quality of life. While traditional treatments exist, many patients choose complementary therapies to manage their symptoms and boost their general well-being. Among these methods, massage therapy stands out as a widely adopted treatment for its capacity to reduce joint pain and enhance mobility. In this extensive examination, we dig into the nuanced advantages of massage therapy in the context of arthritis care, providing light on its physiological underpinnings and practical applications.

Understanding Arthritis and its influence: Before diving into the therapeutic world of massage, it's necessary to appreciate the subtleties of arthritis and its diverse influence on individuals. Arthritis comprises a variety of disorders, including osteoarthritis and rheumatoid arthritis, each marked by inflammation inside the joints. Beyond physical discomfort, arthritis can limit movement, upset sleep habits, and even damage mental well-being, making it vital to embrace holistic methods to its care.

The Therapeutic Power of Touch: At the core of massage therapy is the tremendous healing power of touch. Unlike traditional therapies that solely target symptoms, massage therapy offers a comprehensive approach, treating both physical and mental elements of arthritis care. Through expert manipulation of soft tissues, massage therapists may enhance blood flow, reduce muscular tension, and promote relaxation, ultimately delivering respite from the agony of arthritis.

Enhancing Blood Circulation and Joint Mobility: Central to the success of massage treatment in arthritis care is its capacity to promote blood circulation and joint mobility. By applying mild pressure and rhythmic motions to problematic regions, massage therapists can increase the passage of blood and nutrients to inflammatory joints, boosting healing and reducing stiffness. This enhanced circulation not only alleviates discomfort but also increases joint flexibility, enabling persons to move more freely and engage in daily activities with more ease.

Alleviating Pain and Muscle strain: One of the most significant benefits of massage treatment for arthritis sufferers is its power to ease pain and muscle strain. Through focused methods such as kneading, compression, and friction, massage therapists can relieve tension in surrounding muscles, relieving the burden on inflammatory joints. Moreover, the release of endorphins, the body's natural painkillers, during massage adds to pain reduction and creates a sense of well-being, delivering reprieve from the persistent agony associated with arthritis.

Exploring Different Massage Modalities: Massage therapy comprises a varied variety of modalities, each giving unique advantages for arthritis management. From Swedish massage, typified by long, flowing strokes, to deep tissue massage, which targets deeper layers of muscle and connective tissue, individuals have a myriad of alternatives to meet their tastes and requirements. Moreover, specialist methods such as myofascial release and trigger point treatment can give focused relief for specific regions affected by arthritis, further boosting the efficiency of massage as a therapeutic intervention.

Professional vs. Self-Massage Techniques:
While accessing the skills of a professional massage therapist is best for thorough therapy, individuals may also harness the advantages of massage through self-care approaches. Learning basic self-massage exercises and employing products such as foam rollers and massage balls can empower individuals to manage their symptoms proactively and include therapeutic touch into their everyday routines. Whether having a professional massage or practicing self-care at home, the key lies in consistency and awareness, allowing for prolonged alleviation and better well-being over time.

Conclusion: In the arena of arthritis care, where comfort can sometimes feel elusive, massage therapy emerges as a beacon of hope, bringing substantial benefits for both body and mind.

Through its potential to enhance blood circulation, reduce pain, and promote relaxation, massage therapy serves as a helpful supplement to traditional therapies, allowing individuals to retake control over their health and vitality. As we continue to discover the nuances of this ancient healing technique, let us embrace the therapeutic power of touch and go on a path towards holistic wellbeing in the face of arthritis.

REMEDY FIVE

Acupuncture, an ancient practice rooted in traditional Chinese medicine, stands as a beacon of hope for individuals seeking alternative avenues to manage arthritis discomfort. This time-honored technique revolves around the delicate insertion of ultra-thin needles into strategic points on the body, aiming to harmonize the flow of vital energy, known as qi, and stimulate the body's innate healing mechanisms.

At the heart of acupuncture lies the belief in the interconnectedness of the body's various systems, as understood through the lens of traditional Chinese medicine. According to this paradigm, disruptions or blockages in the flow of qi along pathways called meridians can manifest as physical ailments, including arthritis pain. By strategically placing needles along these meridians, acupuncturists endeavor to restore balance and alleviate discomfort.

Research into the efficacy of acupuncture for arthritis pain has yielded promising results, offering a glimmer of hope to those grappling with the daily challenges of joint inflammation. Studies suggest that acupuncture may trigger the release of endorphins, the body's natural pain-relieving chemicals, thereby providing relief from discomfort. Furthermore, acupuncture sessions may promote relaxation and reduce stress levels, which can exacerbate arthritis symptoms.

Beyond its potential analgesic effects, acupuncture holds profound implications for holistic well-being, transcending the mere alleviation of physical pain. Many individuals report experiencing a profound sense of calm and rejuvenation during and after acupuncture sessions, attributing these sensations to the restoration of energetic balance within the body. In this way, acupuncture serves not only as a therapeutic intervention but also as a conduit for reconnecting with one's inner equilibrium.

One of the key strengths of acupuncture lies in its personalized approach to treatment, tailored to the unique needs and experiences of each individual. During an acupuncture session, a skilled practitioner will conduct a thorough assessment of the patient's condition, taking into account factors such as the location and severity of joint pain, as well as any underlying health concerns. This individualized approach allows for targeted interventions that address the root causes of arthritis discomfort, rather than merely masking symptoms.

Furthermore, acupuncture encompasses a spectrum of techniques and modalities, allowing for flexibility and adaptation to suit the preferences and sensitivities of diverse patients. From traditional needle insertion to non-invasive methods such as acupressure and electroacupuncture, practitioners can customize treatment protocols to align with the comfort levels and therapeutic goals of their clients. This versatility underscores the inclusive nature of acupuncture, welcoming individuals of all ages and backgrounds to explore its potential benefits.

In addition to its role in pain management, acupuncture holds promise as a complementary therapy for enhancing overall joint health and mobility. By promoting circulation and reducing inflammation, acupuncture may support the preservation of cartilage and joint function, thereby mitigating the progression of arthritis over time. Integrating acupuncture into a comprehensive wellness regimen, alongside other modalities such as exercise, dietary modifications, and stress management techniques, can foster a synergistic approach to managing arthritis and optimizing quality of life.

While the scientific understanding of acupuncture's mechanisms of action continues to evolve, its enduring popularity and anecdotal success stories speak to its profound impact on countless individuals worldwide. Beyond the realm of clinical research, acupuncture embodies a rich tapestry of cultural heritage and wisdom, passed down through generations as a testament to the enduring power of healing touch. As we continue to explore the frontiers of integrative medicine, acupuncture stands as a timeless reminder of the interconnectedness of mind, body, and spirit in the pursuit of wellness.

REMEDY SIX

Heat Therapy for Arthritis Relief: Unlocking the Power of Warmth

Arthritis, with its persistent hold on joints, often leaves persons seeking for effective strategies to ease discomfort and promote mobility. Among the arsenal of natural therapies, heat therapy appears as a soothing companion, giving a combination of relaxation, flexibility, and pain relief. Let's go deeper into this relaxing method and explore its therapeutic advantages for individuals experiencing arthritic troubles.

Understanding Heat Therapy
Heat treatment, also known as thermotherapy, includes the intentional application of warmth to damaged joints, intending to relax muscular tension, enhance flexibility, and alleviate pain. Unlike its counterpart, cold treatment, which is largely focused towards lowering inflammation, heat therapy addresses the stiffness and pain frequently associated with arthritis.

The Science Behind the Heat

At its heart, heat treatment relies on the principle of vasodilation, where heat induces blood vessels to enlarge, permitting greater blood flow to the afflicted region. This spike in circulation distributes important nutrients and oxygen while whisking away metabolic waste products, encouraging tissue regeneration and relieving pain. Moreover, the warmth causes muscular relaxation, relieving tension and boosting range of motion—a wonderful break for individuals battling with tight, achy joints.

Harnessing the Healing Power
Now, let's investigate the numerous routes via which heat treatment might be exploited to give comfort and rejuvenation:

1. Heating Pads: These multipurpose companions deliver focused warmth, allowing folks to gently relieve arthritic joints. Whether draped over shoulders, wrapped around knees, or tucked against the lower back, heating pads give steady heat to reduce discomfort and encourage relaxation. Opt for electric heating pads for variable temperature settings or adopt microwavable kinds for on-the-go comfort.

2. Warm Towels: Simple yet effective, warm towels give a cost-efficient manner of engaging in heat treatment. Easily available in most households, they may be heated in a microwave or submerged in hot water before being gently placed to achy joints. Not only can they give rapid comfort, but they also stimulate relaxation, making them an excellent addition to one's arthritis management toolset.

3. Warm Baths: A delightful soak in a warm bath acts as a therapeutic getaway, melting away stress and soothing aching joints. Adding Epsom salts or essential oils to the water enriches the experience, infusing it with extra benefits like as muscle relaxation and stress alleviation. However, it's crucial to ensure that the water temperature stays moderately warm, avoiding extremes that may cause inflammation or pain.

4. Electric Blankets: Embracing persons in a cocoon of warmth, electric blankets give prolonged heat treatment throughout the night, supporting peaceful sleep and reducing morning stiffness. With changeable settings adapting to individual tastes, they provide a personalized

option for people seeking ongoing respite from arthritic problems.

Incorporating Heat Therapy into Daily Routine
While heat treatment offers tremendous potential in relieving arthritic stiffness, its success rests on constant and thoughtful incorporation into one's daily routine. Here are some practical strategies for maximizing its benefits:

- Timing Matters: Incorporate heat treatment during times of heightened discomfort, such as upon awakening or after lengthy periods of inactivity. By preemptively treating stiffness and discomfort, folks may restart their day on a more pleasant note.

- Moderation is Key: While warmth can perform wonderfully for arthritic joints, excessive heat exposure may be harmful. Aim for sessions lasting 15-20 minutes at a time, enabling the body to receive the advantages without risking overheating or skin irritation.

- Combine with Movement: Pairing heat treatment with mild stretching exercises can boost its benefits, improving flexibility and promoting joint mobility. Consider introducing easy stretches or yoga positions into your regimen to capitalize on the synergistic interaction between warmth and movement.

- Listen to Your Body: Pay close attention to how your body responds to heat treatment, modifying the time and intensity of sessions accordingly. It's crucial to achieve a balance between comfort and efficacy, adjusting your strategy to meet your specific needs and preferences.

In the hunt for arthritis treatment, heat therapy emerges as a dependable partner, giving warmth, comfort, and regeneration to weary joints. By embracing its therapeutic effects and incorporating it intelligently into one's daily routine, individuals may engage on a path towards greater comfort, flexibility, and general well-being. So, let the calming embrace of warmth guide you on your journey to rheumatic wellbeing, one comforting session at a time.

REMEDY SEVEN

Epsom Salt Soaks: A Soothing Remedy for Arthritis Relief

Living with arthritis can be challenging, but incorporating natural remedies into your routine can offer much-needed relief. One such remedy that has gained popularity for its soothing effects is Epsom salt soaks. This simple yet effective therapy involves soaking in a warm bath infused with Epsom salt, harnessing the power of magnesium sulfate to ease arthritis symptoms. Let's dive deeper into the science behind this time-honored remedy and explore how it can alleviate your discomfort.

Understanding Epsom Salt: Before we delve into its therapeutic benefits, let's unravel the mystery behind Epsom salt. Contrary to its name, Epsom salt is not your typical table salt. It derives its name from the town of Epsom in England, where it was first discovered in natural mineral springs. Chemically known as magnesium sulfate, Epsom salt is a compound composed of magnesium, sulfur, and oxygen. While it resembles traditional salt in appearance, its composition and properties set it apart as a versatile remedy for various ailments, including arthritis.

The Role of Magnesium: One of the key components of Epsom salt is magnesium, a mineral crucial for numerous bodily functions, including muscle and nerve function, energy production, and bone health. Individuals with arthritis often exhibit lower levels of magnesium in their bodies, which can contribute to muscle stiffness, inflammation, and pain. By soaking in an Epsom salt bath, you provide your body with a readily absorbable form of magnesium, replenishing depleted stores and promoting relaxation of tense muscles.

Sulfate's Healing Touch: In addition to magnesium, Epsom salt contains sulfate, another essential nutrient with therapeutic properties. Sulfate plays a vital role in detoxification pathways within the body, aiding in the elimination of toxins and metabolic waste products. For individuals with arthritis, sulfate can help alleviate inflammation by supporting the body's natural detoxification processes. By immersing yourself in an Epsom salt soak, you not only absorb magnesium but also benefit from sulfate's anti-inflammatory effects, providing relief from arthritis-related discomfort.

The Science Behind Epsom Salt Soaks: The efficacy of Epsom salt soaks in relieving arthritis symptoms stems from their ability to modulate inflammatory pathways and promote muscle relaxation. When dissolved in warm water, Epsom salt releases magnesium ions that are absorbed through the skin, a process known as transdermal absorption. These magnesium ions penetrate deep into the tissues, where they interact with receptors involved in muscle contraction and relaxation. By facilitating the influx of calcium into muscle cells, magnesium promotes muscle relaxation, easing the tension and stiffness commonly associated with arthritis.

Reducing Inflammation: In addition to its muscle-relaxing properties, Epsom salt can help combat inflammation, a hallmark feature of arthritis. Sulfate, the other component of Epsom salt, plays a crucial role in this regard. Studies have shown that sulfate ions can inhibit the activity of pro-inflammatory cytokines, molecules that contribute to the inflammatory response in arthritis. By dampening inflammation, Epsom salt soaks can provide significant relief from pain and swelling, allowing individuals with arthritis to enjoy greater mobility and comfort.

Optimizing Your Epsom Salt Soak: To reap the full benefits of Epsom salt therapy, it's essential to use the proper technique and dosage. Begin by filling your bathtub with warm water, ensuring that it's comfortably hot but not scalding. Add one to two cups of Epsom salt to the bathwater, stirring gently to ensure thorough dissolution. The ideal concentration of Epsom salt may vary depending on individual preferences and sensitivity, so feel free to adjust the amount accordingly.

Duration and Frequency: When it comes to soaking in an Epsom salt bath, timing is key. Aim to immerse yourself in the warm water for at least 15 to 20 minutes to allow for adequate absorption of magnesium and sulfate. During this time, focus on relaxation, deep breathing, and mindfulness, allowing the therapeutic effects of the bath to take hold. For optimal results, consider incorporating Epsom salt soaks into your regular self-care routine, whether it's once a week or more frequently as needed.

Enhancing the Experience: While Epsom salt baths offer undeniable benefits on their own, you can amplify their therapeutic effects by incorporating additional elements into your soak. Experiment with aromatic essential oils such as lavender or eucalyptus, known for their calming and anti-inflammatory properties. You can also add dried herbs or flower petals to infuse your bath with natural fragrance and visual appeal. By customizing your Epsom salt soak to suit your preferences, you can transform it into a luxurious and rejuvenating experience.

Precautions and Considerations: While Epsom salt baths are generally safe for most individuals, it's essential to exercise caution, particularly if you have certain medical conditions or sensitivities. If you have open wounds, infections, or skin conditions such as eczema, consult with your healthcare provider before using Epsom salt soaks. Additionally, individuals with kidney disease or impaired renal function should exercise caution when using magnesium-containing products, as excessive intake can exacerbate their condition.

Epsom salt soaks offer a simple yet effective remedy for arthritis relief, harnessing the therapeutic properties of magnesium sulfate to ease pain, inflammation, and muscle tension. By incorporating regular Epsom salt baths into your self-care routine, you can experience the soothing benefits of this time-honored remedy and reclaim control over your arthritis symptoms. Remember to customize your soak to suit your preferences, experiment with different additives, and prioritize relaxation to maximize the therapeutic effects. With dedication and consistency, Epsom salt therapy can become a valuable tool in your arsenal against arthritis, helping you lead a more comfortable and fulfilling life.

REMEDY EIGHT

Harnessing the Healing Power of Tai Chi for Arthritis Relief

Arthritis, a condition characterized by joint inflammation and stiffness, can significantly impact one's quality of life. While traditional treatments like medication and physical therapy are commonly prescribed, there's a growing interest in alternative therapies that offer holistic benefits. Among these, Tai Chi emerges as a gentle yet powerful contender, seamlessly blending movement, mindfulness, and breathwork to alleviate arthritis symptoms and promote overall well-being.

Understanding Tai Chi:
At its core, Tai Chi is a centuries-old Chinese martial art that has evolved into a graceful, meditative exercise. Unlike high-impact activities that may exacerbate joint pain, Tai Chi's slow, deliberate movements prioritize fluidity over force, making it suitable for individuals of all ages and fitness levels. By emphasizing proper posture and controlled

breathing, Tai Chi cultivates a mind-body connection that fosters relaxation and resilience.

The Science Behind Tai Chi:
Research into the therapeutic effects of Tai Chi on arthritis has yielded promising results. A meta-analysis published in the Journal of Rheumatology concluded that Tai Chi interventions significantly reduced pain and improved physical function in individuals with various forms of arthritis. This can be attributed to several factors, including increased joint flexibility, enhanced muscle strength, and heightened proprioception—the body's awareness of its position in space.

Benefits Beyond the Joints:
Beyond its direct impact on arthritis symptoms, Tai Chi offers a plethora of additional benefits that contribute to overall health and well-being. Regular practice has been linked to improved balance and coordination, which are particularly crucial for individuals with arthritis who may be at an increased risk of falls. Furthermore, Tai Chi has been shown to reduce stress levels and promote relaxation, which can help alleviate the

psychological burden often associated with chronic pain conditions.

Empowering Self-Management:
One of the most empowering aspects of Tai Chi is its emphasis on self-management and self-care. Unlike passive treatments where individuals rely solely on external interventions, Tai Chi empowers participants to take an active role in their healing journey. By cultivating mindfulness and body awareness, individuals develop a deeper understanding of their physical limitations and learn to move with greater ease and efficiency.

Incorporating Tai Chi into Daily Life:
The beauty of Tai Chi lies in its accessibility and adaptability. Whether performed in a class setting or practiced independently at home, Tai Chi can easily be integrated into daily routines. For those with arthritis, it's essential to start slowly and listen to the body's signals. Gradually increasing the duration and intensity of practice allows for steady progress while minimizing the risk of injury.

Creating a Supportive Environment:

For individuals with arthritis, finding a supportive community can make all the difference in maintaining a consistent Tai Chi practice. Joining a local Tai Chi group or participating in online communities provides opportunities for camaraderie, shared experiences, and ongoing motivation. Additionally, partnering with a qualified instructor who understands the unique needs of individuals with arthritis ensures safe and effective guidance throughout the journey.

The Journey Towards Healing:
Ultimately, embracing Tai Chi as a complementary therapy for arthritis is not merely about symptom management but about embracing a holistic approach to health and wellness. By nurturing the body, mind, and spirit in unison, Tai Chi offers a pathway towards greater resilience, vitality, and joy in the face of arthritis's challenges. With dedication, patience, and an open heart, individuals can embark on a transformative journey towards healing and wholeness through the timeless practice of Tai Chi.

In conclusion, Tai Chi stands as a beacon of hope for those navigating the complexities of arthritis. With its gentle yet profound impact on physical, emotional, and spiritual well-being, Tai Chi transcends the limitations of conventional treatments to offer a holistic path towards healing and empowerment. As we embrace the ancient wisdom of Tai Chi and integrate it into our modern lives, we unlock the potential for profound transformation and renewed vitality amidst the journey of arthritis.

REMEDY NINE

Exploring the Therapeutic Potential of Capsaicin Cream for Arthritis Relief

Arthritis, a prevalent condition affecting millions worldwide, often presents debilitating pain and discomfort, significantly impacting one's quality of life. While conventional treatments offer relief, many individuals seek alternative remedies to manage their symptoms effectively. Among these alternatives, capsaicin cream, derived from chili peppers, has garnered attention for its potential in alleviating arthritis-related pain. In this comprehensive guide, we delve into the mechanisms, benefits, and application of capsaicin cream as a natural remedy for arthritis.

Understanding Capsaicin:
Before delving into its therapeutic applications, it's essential to understand capsaicin's properties and how they interact with the body. Capsaicin, the active component in chili peppers responsible for their spiciness, possesses unique analgesic properties. When applied topically, capsaicin interacts with sensory nerve endings,

initiating a cascade of events that ultimately modulate pain perception.

Mechanism of Action:
Capsaicin's mechanism of action revolves around its ability to desensitize sensory nerve receptors, specifically those involved in pain transmission. Upon application, capsaicin binds to transient receptor potential vanilloid 1 (TRPV1) receptors, which are abundant in the skin and peripheral nerves. This binding triggers a series of events, including the depletion of neurotransmitters like substance P, responsible for transmitting pain signals to the brain. Consequently, the perception of pain diminishes, providing relief to individuals suffering from arthritis-related discomfort.

Efficacy in Arthritis Management:
Numerous studies have investigated the efficacy of capsaicin cream in arthritis management, with promising results. One notable study published in the "Journal of Rheumatology" demonstrated significant pain reduction in individuals with osteoarthritis following capsaicin cream application. The cream's analgesic effects were attributed to its ability to

modulate pain signaling pathways, offering a non-invasive and well-tolerated option for arthritis relief.

Application and Dosage:

Proper application and dosage are crucial factors influencing the effectiveness of capsaicin cream in arthritis management. Before applying the cream, it's advisable to cleanse the affected area with mild soap and water to remove any debris or oil. Once the skin is dry, a thin layer of capsaicin cream can be gently massaged into the affected joint or area. It's essential to avoid contact with mucous membranes, eyes, and broken or irritated skin to prevent potential irritation.

Regarding dosage, it's recommended to start with a low concentration of capsaicin cream, gradually increasing the concentration based on individual tolerance and response. Typically, creams containing 0.025% to 0.075% capsaicin are used for arthritis relief, with higher concentrations reserved for chronic pain conditions.

Potential Side Effects:

While generally well-tolerated, capsaicin cream may cause mild side effects, particularly during the initial application phase. These side effects, including temporary burning or stinging sensations at the application site, are transient and usually diminish with continued use. However, individuals with sensitive skin or underlying skin conditions should exercise caution when using capsaicin cream and perform a patch test before widespread application.

Safety Precautions:
To ensure safe and effective use, certain precautions should be observed when using capsaicin cream. It's essential to wash hands thoroughly after application to avoid accidental contact with sensitive areas. Additionally, avoiding exposure to extreme heat or cold immediately after applying capsaicin cream can minimize the risk of adverse reactions. Individuals with known allergies to chili peppers or previous adverse reactions to capsaicin should refrain from using capsaicin cream or consult a healthcare professional before doing so.

In conclusion, capsaicin cream offers a promising natural remedy for individuals seeking relief from arthritis-related pain and discomfort. Its unique mechanism of action, coupled with its well-established safety profile, makes it a valuable addition to the arsenal of arthritis management strategies. By understanding how capsaicin interacts with the body and following proper application guidelines, individuals can harness its therapeutic potential to enhance their quality of life amidst arthritis challenges.

REMEDY TEN

Nourishing the Joints: Harnessing the Power of Dietary Changes to Alleviate Arthritis Symptoms

Arthritis, a condition marked by inflammation of the joints, can significantly impact one's quality of life. While there are various treatment options available, including medication and physical therapy, adopting dietary changes can also play a crucial role in managing arthritis symptoms. In this section, we delve into the profound impact of dietary choices on arthritis and explore how embracing a wholesome, anti-inflammatory diet can provide relief and promote joint health.

1. Understanding Arthritis and Inflammation:
Before delving into dietary recommendations, it's essential to grasp the connection between arthritis and inflammation. Arthritis encompasses a range of conditions characterized by joint inflammation, stiffness, and pain. Inflammation is the body's natural response to injury or illness, but in conditions like arthritis, it becomes chronic, leading to

ongoing discomfort and tissue damage. By targeting inflammation through dietary interventions, individuals with arthritis can potentially mitigate symptoms and improve overall well-being.

2. The Role of Diet in Arthritis Management:
Dietary choices exert a profound influence on inflammation levels in the body. Certain foods can either fuel inflammation or help dampen it, making dietary modifications a valuable tool in managing arthritis. By focusing on whole, nutrient-dense foods and minimizing consumption of inflammatory culprits, individuals can create an internal environment that supports joint health and reduces discomfort.

3. Embracing an Anti-Inflammatory Diet:
Central to managing arthritis through diet is adopting an anti-inflammatory eating pattern. This involves prioritizing foods that possess anti-inflammatory properties while minimizing those known to promote inflammation. A cornerstone of the anti-inflammatory diet is the emphasis on plant-based foods, including fruits, vegetables, legumes, and whole grains. These

foods are rich in vitamins, minerals, and phytonutrients that possess potent anti-inflammatory effects, helping to soothe joint pain and improve mobility.

4. Fruits and Vegetables: Nature's Anti-Inflammatory Allies:
Fruits and vegetables are nutritional powerhouses that offer a myriad of health benefits, including combating inflammation. Rich in antioxidants such as vitamins C and E, as well as flavonoids and carotenoids, these colorful plant foods help neutralize free radicals and reduce oxidative stress in the body. Additionally, certain fruits like berries and cherries contain compounds with anti-inflammatory properties, making them particularly beneficial for arthritis sufferers. By incorporating a diverse array of fruits and vegetables into daily meals, individuals can harness their anti-inflammatory potential and support joint health.

5. Whole Grains: Fiber-Rich Champions of Joint Health:
Whole grains, such as quinoa, brown rice, and oats, are not only wholesome sources of

complex carbohydrates but also valuable allies in the fight against inflammation. Unlike refined grains, which have been stripped of their fiber and nutrients, whole grains retain their fiber content, which has been linked to reduced inflammation and improved joint function. Fiber helps maintain a healthy gut microbiome, which plays a crucial role in regulating immune function and inflammation. By opting for whole grain alternatives to refined grains, individuals with arthritis can support their joint health while enjoying satisfying and nutritious meals.

6. Lean Proteins: Building Blocks for Stronger Joints:

Protein is essential for tissue repair and muscle maintenance, making it a vital component of an arthritis-friendly diet. However, not all protein sources are created equal, especially when it comes to inflammation. Lean proteins, such as poultry, fish, tofu, and legumes, provide high-quality protein without the added saturated fats found in red and processed meats. Additionally, certain fatty fish like salmon, mackerel, and sardines are rich in omega-3 fatty acids, which have potent anti-inflammatory properties. Incorporating these lean protein sources into meals can help support joint health and reduce arthritis-related inflammation.

7. Steering Clear of Inflammatory Culprits:
In addition to emphasizing anti-inflammatory foods, it's equally important to minimize consumption of inflammatory culprits that can exacerbate arthritis symptoms. Processed foods, refined sugars, and saturated fats are notorious for promoting inflammation in the body. Processed foods often contain high levels of additives, preservatives, and unhealthy fats, which can trigger inflammatory responses. Similarly, excessive intake of refined sugars can lead to spikes in blood sugar levels, contributing to inflammation and oxidative stress. By reducing reliance on processed foods and sugary treats and opting for whole, unprocessed alternatives, individuals can create a dietary environment that supports joint health and overall well-being.

8. The Impact of Lifestyle Factors on Arthritis:
While dietary changes are instrumental in managing arthritis, it's essential to recognize the interconnectedness of lifestyle factors in promoting joint health. Regular physical

activity, stress management techniques, adequate sleep, and maintaining a healthy weight all play integral roles in managing arthritis symptoms and reducing inflammation. By adopting a holistic approach that encompasses dietary modifications alongside lifestyle adjustments, individuals can optimize their health and well-being while living with arthritis.

In conclusion, dietary changes represent a powerful and accessible strategy for managing arthritis symptoms and promoting joint health. By embracing an anti-inflammatory eating pattern rich in fruits, vegetables, whole grains, and lean proteins, individuals can create an internal environment that supports reduced inflammation and improved mobility. Moreover, by steering clear of inflammatory culprits such as processed foods and refined sugars, individuals can further enhance their joint health and overall well-being. When combined with other lifestyle factors such as regular exercise and stress management, dietary modifications can serve as a cornerstone of comprehensive arthritis management. By empowering individuals with the knowledge and tools to make informed dietary choices, we can work towards alleviating the burden of arthritis and enhancing the quality of life for millions worldwide.

CONCLUSION

In wrapping up our exploration of natural remedies for arthritis, it's clear that a holistic approach holds immense promise for those seeking relief from this chronic condition. Through the power of nature's bounty and centuries-old healing practices, we've uncovered a wealth of solutions that offer hope, comfort, and tangible results.

Turmeric, with its vibrant hue and potent curcumin compound, stands as a shining example of nature's anti-inflammatory prowess. Whether enjoyed in culinary creations or consumed as a supplement, turmeric offers a simple yet profound way to combat inflammation and ease the burden of arthritis pain.

Omega-3 fatty acids, found abundantly in fatty fish like salmon and mackerel, offer another avenue for relief. By incorporating these omega-3-rich foods into your diet or supplementing with fish oil, you can help reduce joint pain and stiffness, restoring greater freedom of movement and flexibility.

Ginger, revered for its zesty flavor and medicinal properties, emerges as a versatile ally in the fight against arthritis. From soothing ginger teas to culinary concoctions, this humble root offers potent anti-inflammatory benefits, providing much-needed comfort to achy joints.

But our journey doesn't end there. We've also explored the therapeutic benefits of massage therapy and acupuncture, both of which offer holistic approaches to pain management and healing. By addressing not just the symptoms but the underlying imbalances within the body, these ancient practices offer profound relief and rejuvenation.

Heat therapy and Epsom salt soaks provide additional avenues for relaxation and relief, offering soothing comfort to tired muscles and inflamed joints alike. And let's not forget the gentle yet powerful practice of Tai Chi, which offers a graceful way to improve balance, flexibility, and strength while easing the burden of arthritis symptoms.

For those seeking targeted relief, capsaicin cream offers a potent solution derived from chili peppers. By desensitizing nerve receptors and dulling the perception of pain, this topical treatment provides targeted relief where it's needed most.

And finally, we've emphasized the importance of dietary changes in managing arthritis symptoms. By embracing a diet rich in anti-inflammatory foods such as fruits, vegetables, whole grains, and lean proteins, you can help minimize inflammation and support overall joint health from the inside out.

In closing, the path to managing arthritis naturally is as diverse as it is promising. By harnessing the power of nature's remedies and ancient healing practices, you can take proactive steps towards reclaiming control over your health and well-being. Remember, the journey may have its ups and downs, but with perseverance, patience, and a commitment to holistic wellness, relief is within reach.

100 DIETICIAN APPROVED MEDITERRANEAN ANTI-INFLAMMATORY RECIPES

- **MEDITERRANEAN DIET RECIPES**

These recipes offer a variety of flavors and ingredients that showcase the richness and versatility of the Mediterranean diet while providing essential nutrients and promoting overall health. Enjoy exploring these delicious and nutritious dishes!

1. Mediterranean Quinoa Salad:

   - Ingredients: Quinoa, cherry tomatoes, cucumber, Kalamata olives, feta cheese, red onion, olive oil, lemon juice, fresh herbs (such as parsley or basil).

   - Directions: Cook quinoa according to package instructions. Mix with chopped vegetables, olives, and crumbled feta. Drizzle with olive oil and lemon juice, then toss to combine. Garnish with fresh herbs.

2. Grilled Mediterranean Chicken:

   - Ingredients: Chicken breast, lemon juice, olive oil, garlic, oregano, salt, pepper.

   - Directions: Marinate chicken breast in lemon juice, olive oil, minced garlic, dried oregano, salt, and pepper for at least 30 minutes. Grill until cooked through, then serve with a side of grilled vegetables or Greek salad.

3. Greek Yogurt Parfait:
   - Ingredients: Greek yogurt, honey, mixed berries (such as strawberries, blueberries, and raspberries), granola, chopped nuts (such as almonds or walnuts).
   - Directions: Layer Greek yogurt, honey, mixed berries, granola, and chopped nuts in a glass or bowl to create a parfait. Serve as a nutritious breakfast or snack.

4. Mediterranean Stuffed Peppers:
   - Ingredients: Bell peppers, cooked quinoa, chickpeas, cherry tomatoes, spinach, feta cheese, olive oil, garlic, oregano, salt, pepper.
   - Directions: Cut bell peppers in half and remove seeds. Stuff with a mixture of cooked quinoa, chickpeas, chopped tomatoes, spinach, crumbled feta, minced garlic, olive oil, dried oregano, salt, and pepper. Bake until peppers are tender.

5. Mediterranean Veggie Wrap:

- Ingredients: Whole wheat tortilla, hummus, roasted vegetables (such as eggplant, zucchini, bell peppers), sliced cucumber, cherry tomatoes, feta cheese, olives, fresh herbs (such as parsley or basil).

- Directions: Spread hummus on a whole wheat tortilla. Layer with roasted vegetables, sliced cucumber, cherry tomatoes, crumbled feta, and olives. Add fresh herbs, then wrap tightly.

6. Lemon Garlic Shrimp Pasta:

- Ingredients: Whole wheat pasta, shrimp, olive oil, garlic, lemon juice, cherry tomatoes, spinach, feta cheese, fresh herbs (such as parsley or basil).

- Directions: Cook whole wheat pasta according to package instructions. In a separate pan, sauté shrimp in olive oil with minced garlic until cooked through. Add cooked pasta, lemon juice, halved cherry tomatoes, and spinach to the pan. Toss until combined, then top with crumbled feta and fresh herbs.

7. Mediterranean Chickpea Salad:

- Ingredients: Chickpeas, cucumber, cherry tomatoes, red onion, Kalamata olives, feta cheese, olive oil, lemon juice, fresh herbs (such as parsley or dill), salt, pepper.

- Directions: Mix together drained and rinsed chickpeas, chopped cucumber, halved cherry tomatoes, sliced red onion, halved Kalamata olives, and crumbled feta. Dress with olive oil, lemon juice, chopped herbs, salt, and pepper.

8. Greek Lentil Soup:

- Ingredients: Lentils, vegetable broth, onion, carrot, celery, garlic, diced tomatoes, spinach, lemon juice, olive oil, dried oregano, salt, pepper.

- Directions: Sauté diced onion, carrot, celery, and minced garlic in olive oil until softened. Add rinsed lentils, vegetable broth, diced tomatoes, dried oregano, salt, and pepper. Simmer until lentils are tender. Stir in spinach and lemon juice before serving.

9. Mediterranean Egg Breakfast Skillet:

- Ingredients: Eggs, cherry tomatoes, spinach, red onion, Kalamata olives, feta cheese, olive oil, garlic, dried oregano, salt, pepper.

- Directions: Sauté sliced red onion and minced garlic in olive oil until softened. Add halved cherry tomatoes, chopped spinach, and sliced Kalamata olives to the pan. Crack eggs over the vegetables and sprinkle with crumbled feta, dried oregano, salt, and pepper. Cover and cook until eggs are set.

10. Mediterranean Baked Fish:

- Ingredients: White fish filets (such as cod or tilapia), olive oil, lemon juice, garlic, cherry tomatoes, Kalamata olives, capers, fresh herbs (such as parsley or dill), salt, pepper.

- Directions: Place fish filets in a baking dish. Drizzle with olive oil and lemon juice, then season with minced garlic, halved cherry tomatoes, sliced Kalamata olives, capers, chopped herbs, salt, and pepper. Bake until the fish is cooked through.

11. Mediterranean Stuffed Portobello Mushrooms:

- Ingredients: Portobello mushrooms, quinoa, roasted red peppers, artichoke hearts, feta cheese, spinach, garlic, olive oil, lemon juice, fresh herbs (such as parsley or basil), salt, pepper.

- Directions: Remove stems from portobello mushrooms and scrape out gills. Stuff with a mixture of cooked quinoa, diced roasted red peppers, chopped artichoke hearts, crumbled feta, chopped spinach, minced garlic, olive oil, lemon juice, chopped herbs, salt, and pepper. Bake until mushrooms are tender.

12. Mediterranean Tuna Salad:
   - Ingredients: Canned tuna, cherry tomatoes, cucumber, red onion, Kalamata olives, feta cheese, olive oil, lemon juice, fresh herbs (such as parsley or dill), salt, pepper.
   - Directions: Mix together drained canned tuna, halved cherry tomatoes, diced cucumber, sliced red onion, halved Kalamata olives, crumbled feta, olive oil, lemon juice, chopped herbs, salt, and pepper. Serve on a bed of mixed greens or whole wheat bread.

13. Mediterranean Lentil and Vegetable Soup:
   - Ingredients: Lentils, vegetable broth, onion, carrot, celery, zucchini, diced tomatoes, garlic, olive oil, lemon juice, dried oregano, dried thyme, salt, pepper.
   - Directions: Sauté diced onion, carrot, celery, zucchini, and minced garlic in olive oil until softened. Add rinsed lentils, vegetable broth, diced tomatoes, dried oregano, dried thyme,

salt, and pepper. Simmer until lentils are tender. Stir in lemon juice before serving.

14. Mediterranean Roasted Vegetable Platter:
   - Ingredients: Assorted vegetables (such as eggplant, zucchini, bell peppers, cherry tomatoes, red onion), olive oil, garlic, dried oregano, dried thyme, salt, pepper.
   - Directions: Arrange sliced vegetables on a baking sheet. Drizzle with olive oil and sprinkle with minced garlic, dried oregano, dried thyme, salt, and pepper. Roast in the oven until vegetables are tender and slightly caramelized.

15. Greek Style Baked Eggplant:
   - Ingredients: Eggplant, olive oil, garlic, cherry tomatoes, Kalamata olives, feta cheese, fresh herbs (such as parsley or basil), salt, pepper.
   - Directions: Slice eggplant into rounds and place on a baking sheet. Drizzle with olive oil and sprinkle with minced garlic, halved cherry tomatoes, sliced Kalamata olives, crumbled feta, chopped herbs, salt, and pepper. Bake until the eggplant is tender.

16. Mediterranean Chickpea and Vegetable Stir-fry:

- Ingredients: Chickpeas, bell peppers, zucchini, onion, garlic, cherry tomatoes, Kalamata olives, olive oil, lemon juice, dried oregano, salt, pepper.

- Directions: Sauté sliced bell peppers, diced zucchini, sliced onion, and minced garlic in olive oil until softened. Add drained and rinsed chickpeas, halved cherry tomatoes, halved Kalamata olives, lemon juice, dried oregano, salt, and pepper. Cook until heated through.

17. Mediterranean Cauliflower Rice Pilaf:

- Ingredients: Cauliflower rice, onion, garlic, cherry tomatoes, spinach, pine nuts, olive oil, lemon juice, fresh herbs (such as parsley or dill), salt, pepper.

- Directions: Sauté diced onion and minced garlic in olive oil until softened. Add cauliflower rice and cook until tender. Stir in halved cherry tomatoes, chopped spinach, toasted pine nuts, lemon juice, chopped herbs, salt, and pepper.

18. Mediterranean Baked Falafel:

- Ingredients: Chickpeas, onion, garlic, fresh herbs (such as parsley or cilantro), cumin, coriander, olive oil, lemon juice, tahini, yogurt, cucumber, tomato, pita bread.

- Directions: Blend chickpeas, diced onion, minced garlic, chopped herbs, cumin, coriander, olive oil, and lemon juice in a food processor until smooth. Form into balls and bake until golden brown. Serve with tahini-yogurt sauce, diced cucumber, tomato, and warmed pita bread.

19. Mediterranean Zucchini Noodles with Pesto:

- Ingredients: Zucchini noodles (zoodles), cherry tomatoes, Kalamata olives, pine nuts, olive oil, garlic, basil, Parmesan cheese (optional), lemon juice, salt, pepper.

- Directions: Sauté cherry tomatoes, halved Kalamata olives, and pine nuts in olive oil with minced garlic until tomatoes are softened. Toss with raw zucchini noodles, homemade or store-bought pesto, grated Parmesan cheese (if using), lemon juice, salt, and pepper.

20. Greek Style Baked Cod:

- Ingredients: Cod filets, olive oil, garlic, cherry tomatoes, Kalamata olives, capers, fresh herbs (such as parsley or dill), lemon slices, salt, pepper.

- Directions: Place cod filets in a baking dish. Drizzle with olive oil and sprinkle with minced garlic. Top with halved cherry tomatoes, sliced Kalamata olives, capers, chopped herbs, lemon slices, salt, and pepper. Bake until the fish is cooked through.

21. Mediterranean Chickpea Shakshuka:

- Ingredients: Chickpeas, diced tomatoes, onion, garlic, bell peppers, cumin, paprika, cayenne pepper, eggs, olive oil, fresh herbs (such as parsley or cilantro), salt, pepper.

- Directions: Sauté diced onion, minced garlic, and sliced bell peppers in olive oil until softened. Add chickpeas, diced tomatoes, cumin, paprika, and cayenne pepper. Make wells in the mixture and crack eggs into them. Cover and cook until eggs are set. Garnish with fresh herbs before serving.

22. Mediterranean Roasted Beet and Goat Cheese Salad:

- Ingredients: Beets, mixed greens, goat cheese, walnuts, olive oil, balsamic vinegar, honey, Dijon mustard, salt, pepper.

- Directions: Roast beets until tender, then slice thinly. Toss mixed greens with crumbled goat cheese and chopped walnuts. Whisk together olive oil, balsamic vinegar, honey, Dijon mustard, salt, and pepper to make the dressing. Drizzle over the salad and top with roasted beets.

23. Mediterranean Turkey and Feta Meatballs:

- Ingredients: Ground turkey, feta cheese, garlic, onion, fresh herbs (such as parsley or oregano), lemon zest, olive oil, salt, pepper.

- Directions: Mix together ground turkey, crumbled feta cheese, minced garlic, diced onion, chopped herbs, lemon zest, salt, and pepper. Form into meatballs and bake until cooked through. Serve with a side of Greek yogurt sauce.

24. Mediterranean Lentil and Feta Stuffed Peppers:

- Ingredients: Bell peppers, lentils, onion, garlic, cherry tomatoes, spinach, feta cheese, olive oil, lemon juice, fresh herbs (such as mint or dill), salt, pepper.

- Directions: Cook lentils according to package instructions. Sauté diced onion and minced garlic in olive oil until softened. Mix together cooked lentils, halved cherry tomatoes, chopped spinach, crumbled feta, lemon juice, chopped herbs, salt, and pepper. Stuff into halved bell peppers and bake until peppers are tender.

25. Mediterranean Eggplant and Chickpea Curry:

- Ingredients: Eggplant, chickpeas, onion, garlic, tomatoes, coconut milk, curry powder, turmeric, cumin, coriander, olive oil, fresh cilantro, salt, pepper.

- Directions: Sauté diced onion and minced garlic in olive oil until softened. Add diced eggplant and cook until slightly softened. Stir in drained and rinsed chickpeas, diced tomatoes, coconut milk, curry powder, turmeric, cumin, coriander, salt, and pepper. Simmer until flavors are blended. Garnish with chopped fresh cilantro before serving.

26. Mediterranean Baked Stuffed Squash:

- Ingredients: Acorn squash or butternut squash, quinoa, dried cranberries, almonds, feta cheese, olive oil, garlic, fresh herbs (such as thyme or sage), salt, pepper.

- Directions: Cut squash in half and scoop out seeds. Roast in the oven until tender. Cook quinoa according to package instructions. Mix cooked quinoa with dried cranberries, chopped almonds, crumbled feta, minced garlic, chopped herbs, olive oil, salt, and pepper. Stuff mixture into roasted squash halves and bake until heated through.

27. Greek Style Lamb Meatballs with Tzatziki:

- Ingredients: Ground lamb, onion, garlic, fresh herbs (such as mint or oregano), lemon zest, olive oil, salt, pepper, Greek yogurt, cucumber, lemon juice, dill, garlic.

- Directions: Mix together ground lamb, diced onion, minced garlic, chopped herbs, lemon zest, olive oil, salt, and pepper. Form into meatballs and bake until cooked through. Serve with homemade tzatziki sauce made from Greek yogurt, grated cucumber, lemon juice, chopped dill, minced garlic, salt, and pepper.

28. Mediterranean Stuffed Cabbage Rolls:

- Ingredients: Cabbage leaves, ground turkey or beef, rice, onion, garlic, diced tomatoes, olive oil, lemon juice, fresh herbs (such as parsley or dill), salt, pepper.

- Directions: Blanch cabbage leaves until softened. Cook rice according to package instructions. Sauté diced onion and minced garlic in olive oil until softened. Mix together cooked rice, cooked ground meat, diced tomatoes, lemon juice, chopped herbs, salt, and pepper. Roll mixture into cabbage leaves and bake until heated through.

29. Mediterranean Style Baked Salmon with Lemon and Dill:

- Ingredients: Salmon filets, lemon slices, garlic, fresh dill, olive oil, salt, pepper.

- Directions: Place salmon filets on a baking sheet. Top with lemon slices, minced garlic, chopped fresh dill, olive oil, salt, and pepper. Bake until salmon is cooked through and flakes easily with a fork.

30. Mediterranean Couscous Stuffed Bell Peppers:

- Ingredients: Bell peppers, couscous, chickpeas, cherry tomatoes, cucumber, red onion, Kalamata olives, feta cheese, olive oil, lemon juice, fresh herbs (such as mint or parsley), salt, pepper.

- Directions: Cook couscous according to package instructions. Mix together cooked couscous, drained and rinsed chickpeas, halved cherry tomatoes, diced cucumber, sliced red onion, halved Kalamata olives, crumbled feta, olive oil, lemon juice, chopped herbs, salt, and pepper. Stuff mixture into halved bell peppers and bake until peppers are tender.

31. Mediterranean Chickpea and Spinach Stuffed Portobello Mushrooms:

- Ingredients: Portobello mushrooms, chickpeas, spinach, red onion, garlic, cherry tomatoes, feta cheese, olive oil, lemon juice, fresh herbs (such as parsley or basil), salt, pepper.

- Directions: Remove stems from portobello mushrooms and scrape out gills. Sauté chickpeas, chopped spinach, diced red onion, minced garlic, halved cherry tomatoes, and crumbled feta in olive oil until vegetables are tender. Stuff mixture into mushrooms and bake until mushrooms are cooked through.

32. Mediterranean Style Cauliflower Rice Salad:

- Ingredients: Cauliflower rice, cucumber, cherry tomatoes, red onion, Kalamata olives, feta cheese, olive oil, lemon juice, fresh herbs (such as dill or mint), salt, pepper.

- Directions: Cook cauliflower rice according to package instructions. Mix with diced cucumber, halved cherry tomatoes, sliced red onion, halved Kalamata olives, crumbled feta, olive oil, lemon juice, chopped herbs, salt, and pepper.

33. Mediterranean Shrimp and Zucchini Skewers:

- Ingredients: Shrimp, zucchini, cherry tomatoes, red onion, lemon slices, olive oil, garlic, dried oregano, salt, pepper.

- Directions: Thread shrimp, sliced zucchini, cherry tomatoes, red onion, and lemon slices onto skewers. Brush with olive oil mixed with minced garlic, dried oregano, salt, and pepper. Grill until shrimp are cooked through and vegetables are tender.

34. Mediterranean Style Stuffed Artichokes:

- Ingredients: Artichokes, breadcrumbs, garlic, lemon zest, fresh herbs (such as parsley or thyme), olive oil, salt, pepper.

- Directions: Trim artichokes and remove tough outer leaves. Mix breadcrumbs with minced garlic, lemon zest, chopped herbs, olive oil, salt, and pepper. Stuff breadcrumb mixture between the leaves of the artichokes. Steam or bake until artichokes are tender.

35. Mediterranean Turkey and Eggplant Moussaka:

- Ingredients: Ground turkey, eggplant, onion, garlic, diced tomatoes, tomato paste, cinnamon, nutmeg, olive oil, Greek yogurt, eggs, Parmesan cheese, fresh herbs (such as parsley or oregano), salt, pepper.

- Directions: Sauté ground turkey with diced onion and minced garlic until cooked through. Layer cooked ground turkey and sliced eggplant in a baking dish. Mix diced tomatoes with tomato paste, cinnamon, nutmeg, salt, and pepper. Pour over the turkey and eggplant. Top with a mixture of Greek yogurt, beaten eggs, grated Parmesan cheese, and chopped herbs. Bake until bubbly and golden.

36. Mediterranean Orzo Salad with Grilled Vegetables:

- Ingredients: Orzo pasta, bell peppers, zucchini, eggplant, red onion, cherry tomatoes, feta cheese, olive oil, lemon juice, fresh herbs (such as basil or parsley), salt, pepper.

- Directions: Cook orzo pasta according to package instructions. Grill sliced bell peppers, zucchini, eggplant, and red onion until tender and slightly charred. Chop grilled vegetables and toss with cooked orzo, halved cherry tomatoes, crumbled feta, olive oil, lemon juice, chopped herbs, salt, and pepper.

37. Greek Style Lamb Kabobs with Tzatziki Sauce:

- Ingredients: Lamb cubes, bell peppers, red onion, cherry tomatoes, olive oil, garlic, lemon juice, dried oregano, salt, pepper, Greek yogurt, cucumber, dill, garlic.

- Directions: Marinate lamb cubes in olive oil, minced garlic, lemon juice, dried oregano, salt, and pepper. Thread lamb cubes onto skewers with bell peppers, red onion, and cherry tomatoes. Grill until lamb is cooked to desired doneness. Serve with homemade tzatziki sauce made from Greek yogurt, grated cucumber, chopped dill, minced garlic, salt, and pepper.

38. Mediterranean Chickpea and Spinach Frittata:
   - Ingredients: Eggs, chickpeas, spinach, red onion, garlic, cherry tomatoes, feta cheese, olive oil, salt, pepper.
   - Directions: Sauté diced red onion and minced garlic in olive oil until softened. Add drained and rinsed chickpeas, chopped spinach, halved cherry tomatoes, and crumbled feta. Pour beaten eggs over the mixture and cook until set. Slice and serve warm or at room temperature.

39. Mediterranean Stuffed Squid with Tomato Sauce:
   - Ingredients: Squid tubes, rice, onion, garlic, cherry tomatoes, Kalamata olives, capers, olive oil, lemon juice, fresh herbs (such as parsley or basil), salt, pepper.
   - Directions: Cook rice according to package instructions. Sauté diced onion and minced garlic in olive oil until softened. Mix cooked rice with halved cherry tomatoes, sliced Kalamata olives, capers, lemon juice, chopped

herbs, salt, and pepper. Stuff mixture into cleaned squid tubes and secure ends with toothpicks. Bake in tomato sauce until the squid is tender.

40. Mediterranean Style Baked Stuffed Tomatoes:
- Ingredients: Beefsteak tomatoes, bulgur wheat, pine nuts, raisins, red onion, garlic, fresh herbs (such as mint or parsley), olive oil, lemon juice, salt, pepper.
- Directions: Cut tops off beefsteak tomatoes and scoop out seeds. Mix cooked bulgur wheat with toasted pine nuts, raisins, diced red onion, minced garlic, chopped herbs, olive oil, lemon juice, salt, and pepper. Stuff mixture into tomatoes and bake until tomatoes are softened.

41. Mediterranean Style Stuffed Bell Peppers with Quinoa and Chickpeas:
- Ingredients: Bell peppers, quinoa, chickpeas, cherry tomatoes, red onion, feta cheese, olive oil, lemon juice, fresh herbs (such as parsley or dill), salt, pepper.
- Directions: Cook quinoa according to package instructions. Mix cooked quinoa with drained and rinsed chickpeas, halved cherry

tomatoes, diced red onion, crumbled feta, olive oil, lemon juice, chopped herbs, salt, and pepper. Stuff mixture into halved bell peppers and bake until peppers are tender.

42. Mediterranean Style Baked Cod with Olives and Tomatoes:
   - Ingredients: Cod filets, cherry tomatoes, Kalamata olives, garlic, olive oil, lemon juice, fresh herbs (such as oregano or thyme), salt, pepper.
   - Directions: Place cod filets in a baking dish. Top with halved cherry tomatoes, sliced Kalamata olives, minced garlic, olive oil, lemon juice, chopped herbs, salt, and pepper. Bake until the fish is cooked through and flakes easily with a fork.

43. Mediterranean Roasted Vegetable and Chickpea Buddha Bowl:
   - Ingredients: Assorted roasted vegetables (such as sweet potatoes, cauliflower, and Brussels sprouts), cooked chickpeas, quinoa, baby spinach, tahini dressing (made with tahini, lemon juice, garlic, olive oil, salt, and pepper).
   - Directions: Arrange roasted vegetables, cooked chickpeas, and quinoa in a bowl. Add a

handful of baby spinach. Drizzle with tahini dressing before serving.

44. Greek Style Stuffed Chicken Breast with Spinach and Feta:

- Ingredients: Chicken breast, spinach, feta cheese, garlic, lemon zest, olive oil, dried oregano, salt, pepper.

- Directions: Butterfly chicken breast and stuff with sautéed spinach, crumbled feta, minced garlic, lemon zest, dried oregano, salt, and pepper. Secure with toothpicks and bake until chicken is cooked through.

45. Mediterranean Tabbouleh Salad with Chickpeas and Mint:

- Ingredients: Bulgur wheat, cherry tomatoes, cucumber, red onion, parsley, mint, chickpeas, olive oil, lemon juice, salt, pepper.

- Directions: Cook bulgur wheat according to package instructions and let cool. Mix cooked bulgur with halved cherry tomatoes, diced cucumber, finely chopped red onion, chopped parsley, chopped mint, cooked chickpeas, olive oil, lemon juice, salt, and pepper.

46. Mediterranean Style Lentil Soup with Kale and Lemon:

- Ingredients: Lentils, kale, onion, carrot, celery, garlic, diced tomatoes, vegetable broth, olive oil, lemon zest, fresh herbs (such as thyme or rosemary), salt, pepper.

- Directions: Sauté diced onion, carrot, celery, and minced garlic in olive oil until softened. Add lentils, diced tomatoes, vegetable broth, lemon zest, chopped herbs, salt, and pepper. Simmer until lentils are tender. Stir in chopped kale and cook until wilted before serving.

47. Mediterranean Style Shakshuka with Feta and Olives:

- Ingredients: Eggs, diced tomatoes, red bell pepper, onion, garlic, Kalamata olives, feta cheese, olive oil, paprika, cumin, fresh herbs (such as parsley or cilantro), salt, pepper.

- Directions: Sauté diced onion, red bell pepper, and minced garlic in olive oil until softened. Add diced tomatoes, paprika, cumin, salt, and pepper. Simmer until the sauce thickens. Make wells in the sauce and crack eggs into them. Top with crumbled feta and halved Kalamata olives. Cover and cook until eggs are set. Garnish with fresh herbs before serving.

48. Mediterranean Style Baked Eggplant Parmesan:
- Ingredients: Eggplant, marinara sauce, mozzarella cheese, Parmesan cheese, breadcrumbs, garlic, olive oil, fresh basil, salt, pepper.
- Directions: Slice eggplant and brush with olive oil. Bake until tender. Layer baked eggplant slices with marinara sauce, mozzarella cheese, grated Parmesan cheese, minced garlic, and chopped fresh basil. Repeat layers and bake until cheese is melted and bubbly.

49. Mediterranean Style Stuffed Zucchini Boats with Turkey and Quinoa:
- Ingredients: Zucchini, ground turkey, cooked quinoa, cherry tomatoes, red onion, garlic, feta cheese, olive oil, lemon juice, fresh herbs (such as dill or mint), salt, pepper.
- Directions: Cut zucchini in half lengthwise and scoop out seeds to create boats. Sauté ground turkey with diced cherry tomatoes, minced garlic, and chopped red onion until cooked through. Mix cooked quinoa with turkey

mixture, crumbled feta, olive oil, lemon juice, chopped herbs, salt, and pepper. Stuff mixture into zucchini boats and bake until zucchini is tender.

50. Mediterranean Style Baked Stuffed Mushrooms with Spinach and Sun-Dried Tomatoes:

- Ingredients: Large mushrooms, spinach, sun-dried tomatoes, garlic, breadcrumbs, Parmesan cheese, olive oil, fresh herbs (such as thyme or parsley), salt, pepper.

- Directions: Remove stems from mushrooms and scoop out gills. Sauté chopped spinach, minced garlic, chopped sun-dried tomatoes, breadcrumbs, grated Parmesan cheese, olive oil, chopped herbs, salt, and pepper. Stuff mixture into mushroom caps and bake until mushrooms are tender and filling is golden brown.

• ANTI-INFLAMMATORY DIET RECIPES

These recipes are not only delicious but also packed with anti-inflammatory ingredients to support overall health and well-being, especially for individuals managing conditions like arthritis. Enjoy.

1. Salmon and Quinoa Salad with Avocado Dressing:

   - Ingredients: Grilled salmon filets, cooked quinoa, mixed greens, cherry tomatoes, cucumber, avocado, olive oil, lemon juice, garlic, fresh dill, salt, pepper.

   - Directions: Arrange mixed greens on a plate and top with cooked quinoa, grilled salmon, sliced cherry tomatoes, and diced cucumber. Blend avocado, olive oil, lemon juice, minced garlic, chopped dill, salt, and pepper to make a creamy dressing. Drizzle over the salad.

2. Turmeric Chickpea Curry:

   - Ingredients: Chickpeas, onion, garlic, ginger, tomatoes, coconut milk, turmeric, cumin, coriander, cinnamon, cayenne pepper, olive oil, fresh cilantro, salt, pepper.

   - Directions: Sauté diced onion, minced garlic, and grated ginger in olive oil until softened. Add diced tomatoes, drained and rinsed chickpeas, coconut milk, and spices. Simmer until flavors meld. Serve over brown rice or quinoa, garnished with fresh cilantro.

3. Roasted Vegetable and Lentil Salad:
   - Ingredients: Mixed roasted vegetables (such as bell peppers, zucchini, eggplant), cooked lentils, baby spinach, red onion, feta cheese, olive oil, balsamic vinegar, Dijon mustard, honey, salt, pepper.
   - Directions: Toss roasted vegetables with cooked lentils, baby spinach, sliced red onion, and crumbled feta. Whisk together olive oil, balsamic vinegar, Dijon mustard, honey, salt, and pepper to make a dressing. Drizzle over the salad.

4. Stuffed Bell Peppers with Turkey and Quinoa:
   - Ingredients: Bell peppers, ground turkey, cooked quinoa, onion, garlic, diced tomatoes, spinach, feta cheese, olive oil, Italian seasoning, salt, pepper.
   - Directions: Cut the tops off bell peppers and remove seeds. Sauté ground turkey with diced onion and minced garlic until cooked through.

Stir in cooked quinoa, diced tomatoes, chopped spinach, crumbled feta, olive oil, Italian seasoning, salt, and pepper. Stuff mixture into bell peppers and bake until peppers are tender.

5. Lemon Herb Baked Chicken with Roasted Vegetables:
   - Ingredients: Chicken breasts, lemon zest, fresh herbs (such as thyme or rosemary), garlic, olive oil, mixed vegetables (such as carrots, Brussels sprouts, and sweet potatoes), salt, pepper.
   - Directions: Marinate chicken breasts in lemon zest, minced garlic, chopped herbs, olive oil, salt, and pepper. Bake until cooked through. Toss mixed vegetables with olive oil, salt, and pepper. Roast until tender. Serve chicken with roasted vegetables.

6. Mediterranean Chickpea and Kale Salad:
   - Ingredients: Chickpeas, kale, cherry tomatoes, cucumber, red onion, Kalamata olives, feta cheese, olive oil, lemon juice, garlic, dried oregano, salt, pepper.
   - Directions: Massage chopped kale with olive oil and lemon juice until tender. Toss with drained and rinsed chickpeas, halved cherry

tomatoes, diced cucumber, sliced red onion, halved Kalamata olives, crumbled feta, minced garlic, dried oregano, salt, and pepper.

7. Quinoa and Black Bean Stuffed Sweet Potatoes:
   - Ingredients: Sweet potatoes, cooked quinoa, black beans, bell peppers, corn, red onion, avocado, lime juice, cilantro, olive oil, cumin, chili powder, salt, pepper.
   - Directions: Bake sweet potatoes until tender. Mix cooked quinoa with black beans, diced bell peppers, corn, diced red onion, chopped avocado, lime juice, chopped cilantro, olive oil, cumin, chili powder, salt, and pepper. Stuff mixture into sweet potatoes.

8. Ginger Turmeric Carrot Soup:
   - Ingredients: Carrots, onion, garlic, ginger, turmeric, coconut milk, vegetable broth, olive oil, lemon juice, fresh cilantro, salt, pepper.
   - Directions: Sauté diced onion, minced garlic, grated ginger, and turmeric in olive oil until fragrant. Add chopped carrots, coconut milk, and vegetable broth. Simmer until carrots are tender. Blend until smooth. Stir in lemon juice, chopped cilantro, salt, and pepper.

9. Sautéed Spinach and Mushroom Quinoa Bowl:

   - Ingredients: Cooked quinoa, baby spinach, mushrooms, garlic, olive oil, lemon zest, pine nuts, feta cheese, salt, pepper.

   - Directions: Sauté sliced mushrooms and minced garlic in olive oil until golden. Add baby spinach and cook until wilted. Toss with cooked quinoa, lemon zest, toasted pine nuts, crumbled feta, salt, and pepper.

10. Baked Halibut with Tomato and Olive Salsa:

   - Ingredients: Halibut filets, cherry tomatoes, Kalamata olives, red onion, garlic, olive oil, lemon juice, fresh parsley, salt, pepper.

   - Directions: Season halibut filets with salt, pepper, and olive oil. Bake until cooked through. Mix halved cherry tomatoes, chopped Kalamata olives, diced red onion, minced garlic, olive oil, lemon juice, chopped parsley, salt, and pepper to make a salsa. Serve halibut with salsa on top.

11. Cauliflower and Chickpea Curry:

- Ingredients: Cauliflower, chickpeas, onion, garlic, ginger, tomatoes, coconut milk, turmeric, cumin, coriander, paprika, olive oil, fresh cilantro, salt, pepper.

- Directions: Sauté diced onion, minced garlic, and grated ginger in olive oil until softened. Add diced tomatoes, drained and rinsed chickpeas, cauliflower florets, coconut milk, and spices. Simmer until the cauliflower is tender. Garnish with chopped cilantro before serving.

12. Stuffed Portobello Mushrooms with Quinoa and Kale:

- Ingredients: Portobello mushrooms, quinoa, kale, onion, garlic, sun-dried tomatoes, pine nuts, olive oil, lemon juice, fresh basil, salt, pepper.

- Directions: Remove stems from portobello mushrooms and scrape out gills. Cook quinoa according to package instructions. Sauté chopped kale, diced onion, minced garlic, chopped sun-dried tomatoes, and toasted pine nuts in olive oil until kale is wilted. Mix with cooked quinoa, lemon juice, chopped basil, salt, and pepper. Stuff mixture into mushrooms and bake until mushrooms are tender.

13. Mediterranean Style Grilled Lamb Kebabs with Yogurt Sauce:

- Ingredients: Lamb cubes, bell peppers, red onion, cherry tomatoes, olive oil, garlic, lemon juice, dried oregano, salt, pepper, Greek yogurt, cucumber, mint, garlic.

- Directions: Marinate lamb cubes in olive oil, minced garlic, lemon juice, dried oregano, salt, and pepper. Thread lamb cubes onto skewers with bell peppers, red onion, and cherry tomatoes. Grill until lamb is cooked to desired doneness. Serve with a side of Greek yogurt sauce made from Greek yogurt, grated cucumber, chopped mint, minced garlic, salt, and pepper.

14. Mediterranean Style Baked Cod with Lemon and Herbs:

- Ingredients: Cod filets, lemon slices, garlic, fresh parsley, fresh dill, olive oil, salt, pepper.

- Directions: Place cod filets on a baking sheet. Top with lemon slices, minced garlic, chopped parsley, chopped dill, olive oil, salt, and pepper. Bake until the fish is cooked through and flakes easily with a fork.

15. Roasted Beet and Quinoa Salad with Arugula and Walnuts:
- Ingredients: Beets, quinoa, arugula, walnuts, goat cheese, olive oil, balsamic vinegar, Dijon mustard, honey, salt, pepper.
- Directions: Roast beets until tender, then dice. Cook quinoa according to package instructions. Toss cooked quinoa with diced roasted beets, arugula, chopped walnuts, crumbled goat cheese, olive oil, balsamic vinegar, Dijon mustard, honey, salt, and pepper.

16. Stuffed Acorn Squash with Wild Rice and Cranberries:
- Ingredients: Acorn squash, wild rice, onion, garlic, celery, dried cranberries, pecans, olive oil, fresh sage, salt, pepper.
- Directions: Cut acorn squash in half and scoop out seeds. Roast until tender. Cook wild rice according to package instructions. Sauté diced onion, minced garlic, and chopped celery in olive oil until softened. Mix cooked wild rice with sautéed vegetables, dried cranberries, chopped pecans, chopped fresh sage, salt, and pepper. Stuff mixture into roasted acorn squash halves.

17. Mediterranean Style Lentil and Vegetable Soup:
   - Ingredients: Lentils, carrot, celery, onion, garlic, diced tomatoes, vegetable broth, olive oil, lemon juice, fresh parsley, salt, pepper.
   - Directions: Sauté diced onion, minced garlic, chopped carrot, and chopped celery in olive oil until softened. Add lentils, diced tomatoes, vegetable broth, lemon juice, salt, and pepper. Simmer until lentils are tender. Stir in chopped fresh parsley before serving.

18. Greek Style Stuffed Bell Peppers with Quinoa and Spinach:
   - Ingredients: Bell peppers, quinoa, spinach, red onion, garlic, diced tomatoes, Kalamata olives, feta cheese, olive oil, lemon juice, dried oregano, salt, pepper.
   - Directions: Cut the tops off bell peppers and remove seeds. Cook quinoa according to package instructions. Sauté chopped spinach, diced red onion, and minced garlic in olive oil until spinach is wilted. Mix cooked quinoa with sautéed vegetables, diced tomatoes, chopped Kalamata olives, crumbled feta, lemon juice, dried oregano, salt, and pepper. Stuff mixture

into bell peppers and bake until peppers are tender.

19. Mediterranean Style Baked Eggplant Parmesan:
   - Ingredients: Eggplant, marinara sauce, mozzarella cheese, Parmesan cheese, breadcrumbs, garlic, olive oil, fresh basil, salt, pepper.
   - Directions: Slice eggplant and brush with olive oil. Bake until tender. Layer baked eggplant slices with marinara sauce, mozzarella cheese, grated Parmesan cheese, minced garlic, and chopped fresh basil. Repeat layers and bake until cheese is melted and bubbly.

20. Spinach and Chickpea Salad with Tahini Dressing:
   - Ingredients: Baby spinach, chickpeas, cucumber, cherry tomatoes, red onion, tahini, lemon juice, garlic, olive oil, water, salt, pepper.
   - Directions: Toss baby spinach with drained and rinsed chickpeas, sliced cucumber, halved cherry tomatoes, and thinly sliced red onion. Whisk together tahini, lemon juice, minced garlic, olive oil, water, salt, and pepper to make

a creamy dressing. Drizzle over the salad before serving.

21. Turmeric Coconut Lentil Soup:
    - Ingredients: Lentils, coconut milk, onion, garlic, ginger, turmeric, cumin, coriander, vegetable broth, olive oil, lemon juice, fresh cilantro, salt, pepper.
    - Directions: Sauté diced onion, minced garlic, and grated ginger in olive oil until softened. Add lentils, coconut milk, turmeric, cumin, coriander, vegetable broth, salt, and pepper. Simmer until the lentils are tender. Stir in fresh cilantro and lemon juice before serving.

22. Miso Glazed Salmon with Roasted Vegetables:
    - Ingredients: Salmon filets, miso paste, honey, soy sauce, garlic, ginger, olive oil, mixed vegetables (such as carrots, broccoli, and bell peppers), sesame seeds, green onions, salt, pepper.
    - Directions: Whisk together miso paste, honey, soy sauce, minced garlic, minced ginger, and olive oil. Brush over salmon filets and bake until cooked through. Toss mixed vegetables with olive oil, salt, and pepper. Roast until

tender. Serve salmon over roasted vegetables and garnish with sesame seeds and sliced green onions.

23. Quinoa Stuffed Bell Peppers with Tofu and Spinach:

- Ingredients: Bell peppers, quinoa, tofu, spinach, onion, garlic, diced tomatoes, Italian seasoning, olive oil, lemon juice, salt, pepper.

- Directions: Cut the tops off bell peppers and remove seeds. Cook quinoa according to package instructions. Sauté diced onion and minced garlic in olive oil until softened. Crumble tofu and add to the pan with spinach, diced tomatoes, cooked quinoa, Italian seasoning, lemon juice, salt, and pepper. Stuff mixture into bell peppers and bake until peppers are tender.

24. Cauliflower Rice Stir-Fry with Shrimp and Vegetables:

- Ingredients: Cauliflower rice, shrimp, mixed vegetables (such as bell peppers, snap peas, and carrots), garlic, ginger, soy sauce, sesame oil, olive oil, green onions, sesame seeds, salt, pepper.

- Directions: Sauté shrimp, mixed vegetables, minced garlic, and grated ginger in olive oil until shrimp are cooked through. Add cauliflower rice and cook until heated through. Stir in soy sauce and sesame oil. Garnish with sliced green onions and sesame seeds before serving.

25. Mediterranean Chickpea and Quinoa Bowl with Lemon Tahini Dressing:

- Ingredients: Cooked quinoa, chickpeas, cucumber, cherry tomatoes, red onion, Kalamata olives, feta cheese, olive oil, lemon juice, tahini, garlic, water, salt, pepper.

- Directions: Toss cooked quinoa with drained and rinsed chickpeas, diced cucumber, halved cherry tomatoes, thinly sliced red onion, chopped Kalamata olives, crumbled feta, olive oil, and lemon juice. Whisk together tahini, minced garlic, water, salt, and pepper to make a creamy dressing. Drizzle over the bowl before serving.

26. Ginger Lime Chicken Lettuce Wraps:

- Ingredients: Chicken breast, lettuce leaves, bell pepper, carrot, cucumber, green onions, garlic, ginger, lime juice, soy sauce, sesame oil, olive oil, cilantro, salt, pepper.

- Directions: Cook chicken breast in olive oil until cooked through. Shred the chicken and toss with minced garlic, grated ginger, lime juice, soy sauce, sesame oil, sliced bell pepper, shredded carrot, sliced cucumber, chopped green onions, and chopped cilantro. Serve wrapped in lettuce leaves.

27. Sweet Potato and Black Bean Chili:

- Ingredients: Sweet potatoes, black beans, diced tomatoes, onion, garlic, chili powder, cumin, paprika, vegetable broth, olive oil, lime juice, fresh cilantro, salt, pepper.

- Directions: Sauté diced onion and minced garlic in olive oil until softened. Add diced sweet potatoes, black beans, diced tomatoes, chili powder, cumin, paprika, vegetable broth, salt, and pepper. Simmer until sweet potatoes are tender. Stir in fresh lime juice and chopped cilantro before serving.

28. Cauliflower and Chickpea Tacos with Avocado Crema:

- Ingredients: Cauliflower florets, chickpeas, taco seasoning, corn tortillas, avocado, Greek yogurt, lime juice, garlic, olive oil, cilantro, red cabbage, salt, pepper.

- Directions: Toss cauliflower florets and chickpeas with taco seasoning and olive oil. Roast until the cauliflower is tender. Mash avocado with Greek yogurt, lime juice, minced garlic, chopped cilantro, salt, and pepper to make a crema. Serve roasted cauliflower and chickpeas in corn tortillas topped with avocado crema and shredded red cabbage.

29. Mediterranean Style Lentil and Quinoa Salad:

- Ingredients: Cooked lentils, cooked quinoa, cucumber, cherry tomatoes, red onion, feta cheese, Kalamata olives, olive oil, lemon juice, fresh parsley, salt, pepper.

- Directions: Toss cooked lentils and quinoa with diced cucumber, halved cherry tomatoes, thinly sliced red onion, crumbled feta, chopped Kalamata olives, olive oil, lemon juice, chopped fresh parsley, salt, and pepper.

30. Spaghetti Squash with Turkey Bolognese Sauce:

- Ingredients: Spaghetti squash, ground turkey, onion, garlic, carrots, celery, diced tomatoes, tomato paste, Italian seasoning, olive oil, fresh basil, salt, pepper.

- Directions: Roast spaghetti squash until tender. Sauté diced onion, minced garlic, diced carrots, and diced celery in olive oil until softened. Add ground turkey and cook until browned. Stir in diced tomatoes, tomato paste, Italian seasoning, salt, and pepper. Simmer until flavors meld. Serve turkey Bolognese sauce over spaghetti squash noodles, garnished with chopped fresh basil.

31. Lemon Garlic Shrimp and Broccoli Stir-Fry:

- Ingredients: Shrimp, broccoli florets, garlic, ginger, lemon zest, olive oil, soy sauce, honey, red pepper flakes, sesame seeds, green onions, salt, pepper.

- Directions: Sauté minced garlic and grated ginger in olive oil until fragrant. Add shrimp and cook until pink. Add broccoli florets, lemon zest, soy sauce, honey, and red pepper flakes. Stir-fry until broccoli is tender. Garnish with sesame seeds and sliced green onions.

32. Moroccan Chickpea Tagine with Apricots and Almonds:

- Ingredients: Chickpeas, onion, garlic, carrots, dried apricots, almonds, vegetable broth, olive oil, ground cinnamon, ground cumin, ground coriander, turmeric, saffron, fresh cilantro, salt, pepper.

- Directions: Sauté diced onion and minced garlic in olive oil until softened. Add diced carrots, drained and rinsed chickpeas, chopped dried apricots, almonds, vegetable broth, and spices. Simmer until carrots are tender. Serve garnished with fresh cilantro.

33. Greek Style Stuffed Portobello Mushrooms with Quinoa and Feta:

- Ingredients: Portobello mushrooms, quinoa, spinach, red bell pepper, red onion, garlic, feta cheese, olive oil, lemon juice, dried oregano, salt, pepper.

- Directions: Remove stems from portobello mushrooms and scrape out gills. Cook quinoa according to package instructions. Sauté chopped spinach, diced red bell pepper, diced red onion, and minced garlic in olive oil until softened. Mix cooked quinoa with sautéed vegetables, crumbled feta, lemon juice, dried oregano, salt, and pepper. Stuff mixture into mushrooms and bake until mushrooms are tender.

34. Turmeric Ginger Carrot Soup:
- Ingredients: Carrots, onion, garlic, ginger, turmeric, coconut milk, vegetable broth, olive oil, lime juice, fresh cilantro, salt, pepper.
- Directions: Sauté diced onion, minced garlic, grated ginger, and turmeric in olive oil until fragrant. Add chopped carrots, coconut milk, vegetable broth, salt, and pepper. Simmer until carrots are tender. Blend until smooth. Stir in fresh lime juice and chopped cilantro before serving.

35. Salmon and Asparagus Foil Packets with Lemon Dill Sauce:
- Ingredients: Salmon filets, asparagus spears, garlic, lemon slices, olive oil, fresh dill, Dijon mustard, Greek yogurt, lemon juice, salt, pepper.
- Directions: Place salmon filets and asparagus spears on a piece of foil. Top with minced garlic, lemon slices, olive oil, and chopped fresh dill. Seal foil packets and bake until salmon is cooked through. Mix Dijon

mustard, Greek yogurt, lemon juice, salt, and pepper to make a sauce. Serve with foil packets.

36. Mediterranean Style Eggplant and Lentil Stew:

- Ingredients: Eggplant, lentils, onion, garlic, diced tomatoes, vegetable broth, olive oil, fresh parsley, lemon zest, cumin, paprika, cinnamon, salt, pepper.

- Directions: Sauté diced onion and minced garlic in olive oil until softened. Add chopped eggplant, lentils, diced tomatoes, vegetable broth, spices, salt, and pepper. Simmer until the eggplant is tender. Stir in chopped fresh parsley and lemon zest before serving.

37. Quinoa and Kale Stuffed Acorn Squash:

- Ingredients: Acorn squash, quinoa, kale, onion, garlic, dried cranberries, pecans, olive oil, balsamic vinegar, maple syrup, fresh thyme, salt, pepper.

- Directions: Cut acorn squash in half and remove seeds. Roast until tender. Cook quinoa according to package instructions. Sauté chopped kale, diced onion, and minced garlic in olive oil until kale is wilted. Mix cooked quinoa with sautéed vegetables, dried cranberries, chopped pecans, balsamic vinegar, maple syrup, fresh thyme, salt, and pepper. Stuff mixture into roasted acorn squash halves.

38. Mediterranean Style Baked Chicken with Artichokes and Olives:
- Ingredients: Chicken thighs, artichoke hearts, Kalamata olives, cherry tomatoes, onion, garlic, olive oil, lemon juice, fresh oregano, salt, pepper.
- Directions: Arrange chicken thighs in a baking dish. Top with quartered artichoke hearts, halved Kalamata olives, halved cherry tomatoes, sliced onion, and minced garlic. Drizzle with olive oil and lemon juice. Sprinkle with chopped fresh oregano, salt, and pepper. Bake until chicken is cooked through.

39. Ginger Turmeric Tofu Stir-Fry with Vegetables:
- Ingredients: Tofu, mixed vegetables (such as bell peppers, broccoli, and snap peas), garlic, ginger, turmeric, soy sauce, sesame oil, olive oil, rice vinegar, green onions, sesame seeds, salt, pepper.
- Directions: Press tofu to remove excess moisture, then cut into cubes. Sauté tofu cubes,

mixed vegetables, minced garlic, and grated ginger in olive oil until vegetables are tender-crisp. Stir in turmeric, soy sauce, sesame oil, and rice vinegar. Garnish with sliced green onions and sesame seeds before serving.

40. Lentil and Vegetable Curry with Coconut Milk:
   - Ingredients: Lentils, mixed vegetables (such as carrots, potatoes, and green beans), onion, garlic, ginger, coconut milk, curry powder, olive oil, lime juice, fresh cilantro, salt, pepper.
   - Directions: Sauté diced onion, minced garlic, and grated ginger in olive oil until softened. Add mixed vegetables, cooked lentils, coconut milk, curry powder, salt, and pepper. Simmer until vegetables are tender. Stir in fresh lime juice and chopped cilantro before serving.

41.Mushroom and Spinach Quinoa Risotto:
   - Ingredients: Quinoa, mushrooms (such as cremini or shiitake), spinach, onion, garlic, vegetable broth, white wine (optional), olive oil, Parmesan cheese (optional), fresh thyme, salt, pepper.
   - Directions: Sauté diced onion and minced garlic in olive oil until softened. Add sliced

mushrooms and cook until browned. Stir in quinoa and cook for a few minutes. Add vegetable broth gradually, stirring frequently until quinoa is cooked and creamy. Fold in chopped spinach, Parmesan cheese (if using), fresh thyme, salt, and pepper.

42. Thai Coconut Curry Soup with Tofu and Vegetables:
   - Ingredients: Tofu, mixed vegetables (such as bell peppers, broccoli, and carrots), coconut milk, red curry paste, vegetable broth, garlic, ginger, lemongrass (optional), lime juice, cilantro, olive oil, salt, pepper.
   - Directions: Sauté diced tofu, mixed vegetables, minced garlic, grated ginger, and chopped lemongrass (if using) in olive oil until vegetables are tender. Stir in red curry paste and cook for a minute. Add coconut milk and vegetable broth. Simmer until flavors meld. Finish with lime juice and chopped cilantro before serving.

43. Turmeric Cauliflower Soup with Coconut Milk:
   - Ingredients: Cauliflower, coconut milk, onion, garlic, ginger, turmeric, vegetable broth,

olive oil, lemon juice, fresh cilantro, salt, pepper.

- Directions: Sauté diced onion, minced garlic, and grated ginger in olive oil until softened. Add chopped cauliflower, turmeric, coconut milk, and vegetable broth. Simmer until the cauliflower is tender. Blend until smooth. Stir in fresh lemon juice, chopped cilantro, salt, and pepper.

44. Sesame Ginger Salmon with Stir-Fried Vegetables:

- Ingredients: Salmon filets, mixed vegetables (such as bell peppers, snap peas, and carrots), garlic, ginger, soy sauce, sesame oil, rice vinegar, honey, olive oil, sesame seeds, green onions, salt, pepper.

- Directions: Marinate salmon filets in a mixture of minced garlic, grated ginger, soy sauce, sesame oil, rice vinegar, and honey. Sear salmon until cooked to desired doneness. Stir-fry mixed vegetables in olive oil until tender-crisp. Serve salmon over stir-fried vegetables, garnished with sesame seeds and sliced green onions.

45. Lentil and Sweet Potato Shepherd's Pie:

- Ingredients: Lentils, sweet potatoes, onion, garlic, carrots, celery, vegetable broth, tomato paste, olive oil, fresh thyme, salt, pepper.

- Directions: Sauté diced onion, minced garlic, chopped carrots, and chopped celery in olive oil until softened. Add cooked lentils, tomato paste, vegetable broth, fresh thyme, salt, and pepper. Simmer until flavors meld. Mash cooked sweet potatoes and spread over the lentil mixture. Bake until bubbly and golden.

46. Miso Glazed Eggplant with Brown Rice:

- Ingredients: Eggplant, brown rice, miso paste, honey, soy sauce, garlic, ginger, olive oil, sesame seeds, green onions, salt, pepper.

- Directions: Slice eggplant and brush with a mixture of miso paste, honey, soy sauce, minced garlic, grated ginger, and olive oil. Roast until tender and caramelized. Serve with cooked brown rice, garnished with sesame seeds and sliced green onions.

47. Roasted Red Pepper and Lentil Soup:

- Ingredients: Red lentils, roasted red peppers, onion, garlic, vegetable broth, coconut milk, olive oil, lemon juice, smoked paprika, cayenne pepper, salt, pepper.

- Directions: Sauté diced onion and minced garlic in olive oil until softened. Add cooked red lentils, chopped roasted red peppers, vegetable broth, coconut milk, smoked paprika, cayenne pepper, salt, and pepper. Simmer until flavors meld. Stir in fresh lemon juice before serving.

48. Mediterranean Stuffed Zucchini Boats:

- Ingredients: Zucchini, quinoa, cherry tomatoes, Kalamata olives, red onion, garlic, feta cheese, olive oil, lemon juice, fresh parsley, dried oregano, salt, pepper.

- Directions: Cut zucchini in half lengthwise and scoop out the flesh to create boats. Cook quinoa according to package instructions. Sauté chopped cherry tomatoes, sliced Kalamata olives, diced red onion, and minced garlic in olive oil until softened. Mix cooked quinoa with sautéed vegetables, crumbled feta, lemon juice, chopped fresh parsley, dried oregano, salt, and pepper. Stuff mixture into zucchini boats and bake until zucchini is tender.

49. Turmeric Coconut Chickpea Curry with Cauliflower Rice:

- Ingredients: Chickpeas, cauliflower, onion, garlic, ginger, coconut milk, turmeric, curry powder, vegetable broth, olive oil, lime juice, fresh cilantro, salt, pepper.

   - Directions: Sauté diced onion, minced garlic, and grated ginger in olive oil until softened. Add drained and rinsed chickpeas, chopped cauliflower, coconut milk, turmeric, curry powder, vegetable broth, salt, and pepper. Simmer until the cauliflower is tender. Stir in fresh lime juice and chopped cilantro before serving over cauliflower rice.

50. Lemon Herb Quinoa Salad with Grilled Chicken:

   - Ingredients: Quinoa, grilled chicken breast, cucumber, cherry tomatoes, red onion, feta cheese, olive oil, lemon juice, fresh basil, fresh mint, fresh parsley, salt, pepper.

   - Directions: Cook quinoa according to package instructions. Toss cooked quinoa with diced grilled chicken breast, diced cucumber, halved cherry tomatoes, thinly sliced red onion, crumbled feta, olive oil, lemon juice, chopped fresh basil, chopped fresh mint, chopped fresh parsley, salt, and pepper.

BONUS: SURE 90 DAYS ARTHRITIS RECOVERY MORNING TEA

Arthritis Remedy: Herbal Paste and Tea Blend
For centuries, herbal remedies have been used to alleviate arthritis symptoms and promote joint health. Among these remedies, a blend of ginger, garlic, lemon, and turmeric has gained attention for its potential therapeutic benefits. When combined and prepared as a paste, this blend can be incorporated into a daily tea regimen to help manage arthritis symptoms effectively.

⇒Ingredients:
- Fresh ginger root
- Garlic cloves
- Lemon
- Turmeric powder

Preparation of the Herbal Paste:
1. Peel and finely chop a piece of fresh ginger root, approximately one inch in size.
2. Peel and crush several cloves of garlic to release their active compounds.

3. Squeeze the juice of one fresh lemon.
4. In a mixing bowl, combine the chopped ginger, crushed garlic, lemon juice, and a tablespoon of turmeric powder.
5. Blend the ingredients together until a smooth paste is formed. Adjust the consistency by adding more lemon juice if necessary.

Storage:
1. Transfer the herbal paste into an airtight container.
2. Store the container in the freezer to preserve the freshness and potency of the ingredients.

Preparation of the Herbal Tea:
1. In the morning, take a tablespoon of the blended herbal paste from the freezer.
2. Add the herbal paste to a pot of water and bring it to a boil.
3. Allow the mixture to simmer for a few minutes to infuse the water with the beneficial compounds of the herbs.
4. Strain the herbal tea into a cup and discard any solids.
5. Optionally, sweeten the tea with honey or maple syrup to taste.

Usage:
1. Drink a cup of the herbal tea daily, preferably in the morning on an empty stomach.
2. Continue this regimen for a duration of at least three months to experience the full benefits of the herbal remedy.

Benefits:
- Ginger: Contains anti-inflammatory compounds that help reduce joint pain and inflammation associated with arthritis.
- Garlic: Exhibits anti-inflammatory and antioxidant properties, which may help alleviate arthritis symptoms and support overall joint health.
- Lemon: Rich in vitamin C and antioxidants, lemon helps boost the immune system and reduce oxidative stress in the body.
- Turmeric: Contains curcumin, a potent anti-inflammatory compound that has been studied for its potential therapeutic effects in arthritis management.

It's important to note that while herbal remedies can provide symptomatic relief for arthritis, they are not a substitute for medical treatment. Individuals with arthritis should consult with a healthcare professional before starting any new treatment regimen, especially if they are taking medications or have underlying health conditions. Additionally, it's essential to monitor for any adverse reactions or interactions with other medications.

By incorporating this herbal remedy into a comprehensive arthritis management plan that includes conventional treatments, dietary modifications, and lifestyle changes, individuals can take proactive steps toward improving their joint health and overall well-being.